# BECKI CONWAY SANDERS
# & JIM & SALLY CONWAY

# What God
# GIVES
# When Life
# TAKES

## The Story of a
## Family in Crisis

INTERVARSITY PRESS
DOWNERS GROVE, ILLINOIS 60515

*InterVarsity Press is the book-publishing division of InterVarsity Christian Fellowship, a student movement active on campus at hundreds of universities, colleges and schools of nursing. For information about local and regional activities, write Public Relations Dept., InterVarsity Christian Fellowship, 6400 Schroeder Rd., P.O. Box 7895, Madison, WI 53707-7895.*

*Distributed in Canada through InterVarsity Press, 860 Denison St., Unit 3, Markham, Ontario L3R 4H1, Canada.*

*All Scripture quotations, unless otherwise indicated, are from the Holy Bible, New International Version. Copyright © 1973, 1978, International Bible Society. Used by permission of Zondervan Bible Publishers.*

*Scripture quotations marked LB are from The Living Bible. Copyright © 1971 by Tyndale House Publishers. Used by permission.*

*The accounts in this book are real, although some names and circumstances have been altered to protect certain individuals.*

*ISBN 0-8308-1714-X*

*Printed in the United States of America*

---

**Library of Congress Cataloging-in-Publication Data**

*Sanders, Becki Conway, 1961-*
    *What God gives when life takes: the story of a family in crisis/*
*Becki Conway Sanders and Jim and Sally Conway.*
        *p.     cm.*
    *ISBN 0-8308-1714-X*
    *1. Sanders, Becki Conway, 1961-     . 2. Christian biography—*
*United States.    3. Cancer—Patients—United States—Biography.*
*4. Cancer—Religious aspects—Christianity.    5. Conway, Jim.*
*6. Conway, Sally.    I. Conway, Jim.    II. Conway, Sally.    III. Title.*
*BR1725.S267A3    1989*
*248.8'6'092—dc20*
    *[B]                                               89-31813*
                                                          *CIP*

---

| 17 | 16 | 15 | 14 | 13 | 12 | 11 | 10 | 9 | 8 | 7 | 6 | 5 | 4 | 3 | 2 | 1 |
| 99 | 98 | 97 | 96 | 95 | 94 | 93 | 92 | 91 | 90 | 89 | | | | | | |

*To my husband, Craig*

*Thanks for being*

> *Creative*
> *Dedicated*
> *Sensitive*
> *Uncompromising*
> *Talented*
> *Intelligent*
> *Spiritually focused*
> *Witty*

*And my closest friend*

# Part I

# GOD'S
# PREPARATION

# 1

# APRIL
# SATURDAY

**W**hat a great day for a track meet! It was a beautiful April Saturday morning. The trees were sprouting their new green leaves. The air was cool and crisp, the sun was bright, and the grass was wet with dew. Even the painted white lines on the gritty cinder track glistened in the morning sun. It felt good to be alive.

I parked the family car along the street and hurried to join the action. I was so anxious to greet my friends that it seemed to take forever to get across the grass playing field to the track.

Several good friends waved and said, "Hi!" Casual acquaintances looked surprised. One of my track teammates hollered, "What are you doing here?"

"Do you think I'd miss the Urbana Invitational?" I replied. "I came to help."

Cars and school buses filled the parking lot, and athletes dressed in their team colors were scattered all over the field, stretching out and running warm-up sprints. Runners paced back and forth, preparing for their events. Others rehearsed relay handoffs, hurdles and starts from the blocks.

I could sense the excitement in the air. As spectators gathered in the stands, coaches offered last-minute pointers to the athletes. The first major track meet of the new season was about to begin.

The announcer welcomed the athletes and their cheering fans, while the nervous runners paced back and forth at the side of the bleachers. The first event was announced, and the participants moved to the starting line, crouching low in the starting blocks. The sun was hotter now, and the morning dampness no longer was on the grass but on the foreheads and backs of the tense runners.

The timers carefully watched for the smoke from the starter's gun to signal the start of the race. The gun fired, muscles released, and the runners sprang out of the blocks. The fans screamed to their favorite runner. The racers, however, only heard the sound of their pounding feet on the track. They were breathing hard as they dug each foot into the cinders. Lifting their knees high and pumping their arms with tightly clenched fists, they focused on the bright orange finish tape that marked their success or failure.

Shouts from the stands grew to a deafening roar. Each of the front runners stretched to cross the finish line first. Their chests were bursting as they gave their last hard kick to break the tape.

The close race was over, and the noise from the crowd subsided. Timers checked their stopwatches and wrote the times on their clipboards. The announcer was already calling for the next event as the first runners moved off the track, gasping for breath, some limping slightly and others holding their aching sides. The next runners positioned themselves in the blocks.

Although I wasn't running in this meet, I was at the track because weeks earlier I had promised my coaches I would help by taking race results to the press booth, timing the events, being a line judge or whatever they needed. Another reason for coming to the meet was that I missed my friends. I had been in the hospital almost a week and was out of school another week recuperating at home. I was eager to tell them about all that had happened to me, and I wanted to see how they'd react.

I felt people staring as I walked through the bleachers. Many recognized me. I had been on the track team as a hurdler, training with the team only weeks earlier. Their eyes spoke their questions, "What happened to you?" "Why are you here at a track meet of all places?" One friend even said, "I really feel sorry for you."

Children gawked and pointed, but their parents quickly reprimanded them. Adults stared, too, but only when they thought my back was turned. I knew they were all looking, though.

Anyway, the meet was going great. Urbana High School was in the top five—not bad for the first competition of the year. I kept busy shuttling the results to the press booth and assisting with timing. Kids from my school warmed up to me as the day went along. Many even began to treat me as if nothing were different. But I knew they all had unanswered questions.

The sun started to slip behind the neighboring housetops as the final events came to an end. The ribbons were awarded and the crowd began to thin. The first track meet of the season was over. So was my first day in public after losing my left leg.

# 2

# HAPPY BIRTHDAY, BECKI

**B**eck the Wreck" is my nickname, and I have always lived up to it. I am very active and athletic—and accident-prone. And so, three days before my fifteenth birthday, I was keeping a doctor's appointment for a dislocated tailbone I'd gotten while cheerleading.

I had seen the doctor three or four times before, but this time I limped into his office. "Now what else is wrong with you?" he asked.

Matter-of-factly, I answered, "Oh . . . well, besides my tailbone, I've got this problem with my left knee. Every once in a while it swells up, I limp around or use crutches for a few days; then the pain goes away. It's been going on for a couple of years."

I explained that two other doctors had told me my ligaments were probably being stressed because I was still growing and very active. They said knee problems were common for girls my age—I'd outgrow it. So I brushed off the matter as I spoke to this doctor.

However, he didn't share my casual attitude and insisted on taking an x-ray. He discovered that the bone above my left knee was three times thicker than normal for a length of about six inches. This really concerned him, and it certainly surprised me. He suggested that we make an appointment with an orthopedist immediately. I never expected this for my fifteenth birthday!

## My Birthday Appointment

Dr. Scott Kline was an orthopedic surgeon new to our local clinic. We knew about him because he attended our church. After the next Sunday morning service, we explained to him what my doctor had found. He urged us to call his office to make an appointment for the next day—my birthday.

After his examination and more x-rays, he told us a large tumor was just above my knee. He suspected some kind of bone lesion but couldn't tell from the x-ray exactly what it was. He wanted me hospitalized for a biopsy as soon as possible. The procedure would include general anesthesia and a two- or three-day hospital stay. During the biopsy he would extract small samples of the tumor tissue to determine its identity.

Dr. Kline was straightforward about the range of possibilities. He gently explained to us that the outcome might be very serious. Probably I would have other surgeries, tests and extensive therapy. I might need a bone graft—or an amputation. Death was even a prospect. He felt the chances were small that the tumor was cancerous, however, and assured me that an amputation probably was remote. As I heard the serious possibilities that day, God gave me an unusual peace about my future.

Somehow, knowing about all the prospects helped me face the unfaceable. During the next weeks and months, in the back of my mind I could hear the echo of "amputation" and "death." Unconsciously, I was considering these possibilities as realities.

When such thoughts came—usually while I was out running or having fun with friends—I vowed to myself and God that I would make the best of it. I dreaded the idea of being a wimp or a whiney, depressed invalid. I did not want to embarrass God who had promised to give me his strength in any circumstance. So, even though these thoughts scared me, every time they appeared, I again gave them to God and asked for his help with whatever happened.

### The First Biopsy
A couple of weeks after I first saw Dr. Kline, I was hospitalized for the biopsy. Everything went as planned, except that during the operation the doctors were surprised to find the tumor much harder than expected. Dr. Kline broke some of his instruments trying to cut samples from it! No conclusions about the growth could be reached during the operation. In fact, it took several days for the sample to be dissolved by the pathologist so that he could analyze it.

The hardness of the tumor seemed a good indication that it might not be cancerous. Many types of bone cancers, such as osteosarcomas and melanomas, are soft. Also, some malignant tumors weaken the bone so that it breaks. Treating the broken bone is often when the cancer is first detected. My thighbone, however, was still very strong.

Dr. Kline remained uncertain about what type of tumor I had, but he felt it probably was not malignant. Of course, he couldn't make any promises. He needed more information. He sent samples of the tumor to other laboratories and consulted with many physicians and pathologists around the United States. The opinions from the consultations were inconclusive. Most doctors agreed, however, that the mysterious tumor didn't seem to be a threat to my health at that time. Dr. Kline decided to observe it over the next months.

Strangely enough, the tumor had actually replaced the bottom of my thighbone—it wasn't just an outside attachment to the bone or a growth in the marrow. The tumor—larger than a lemon—had entirely taken the place of the bottom of my thighbone. As it had grown, it apparently pushed on my knee, causing the swelling, soreness and stiffness that had become an increasing problem during the previous two years.

### Joni—God's Gift

God was preparing me for the future he knew I was to have. While I was recovering from the biopsy, I met Joni Eareckson, who would later be a role model for me. She spoke at two meetings in our city. Sitting in her wheelchair, she used a pen in her mouth to draw a picture. One time she drew a cabin in a beautiful mountain setting. When the drawing was nearly complete, she suddenly ruined the picture with two black lines through either side of the cabin. I wondered, "What is she doing?"

At once she made her point: "Sometimes God allows dark lines to become part of our lives. But he can use those dark experiences to perfect us and help us grow into being the people he wants."

As she continued to speak, she transformed those lines into

beautiful pine trees that served to outline, complement and complete the picture. She talked about her experiences and all that God had taught her as a quadriplegic.

At the time it looked as if my tumor were benign, so I had no idea that I might go through something as life-changing and permanent as her experience. Even so, I was struck by Joni's testimony. It was exciting that God had taken something so awful and turned it into a ministry that glorified God and helped others.

## A Second Biopsy

For a couple of months after the first biopsy, my pain decreased. Dr. Kline thought that drilling into the tumor for the biopsy sample may have relieved some of the pressure. In certain cases drilling has been a prescribed treatment for bone pain. As I recuperated from the biopsy, I worked to get in shape for track again. I was glad to be able to run the hurdles in the spring track season. The pain in my left knee had subsided.

By early fall, however, both of my knees were very painful. I went to Dr. Kline, mainly about my right knee. He ordered a comparative x-ray to look at both knee joints and to check the contrast in the two left knee x-rays taken one year apart. The x-rays disclosed a normal right knee, but the tumor above the left knee was enlarging. During the biopsy, samples had been taken from the outer side of the leg bone; now it looked as if a new part of the tumor was also growing on the inner side of my leg. Fortunately, it still seemed to be contained within the bone wall.

Dr. Kline decided to do a second biopsy. He planned to take out a larger sample of the tumor, anticipating a more definite analysis than from the first biopsy. This time he borrowed the strongest surgical instruments he could locate—from the nearby veterinary medical school! He removed three one-inch-by-one-inch cubes from the growth, hoping that this would give more conclusive results.

Dr. Kline also put my leg in a hip-to-ankle cast to slow me down so my leg could heal. He was afraid that with so much tissue and bone removed, my leg would fracture if I walked on it too soon. The huge cast certainly prevented that!

Again he sent samples to different medical centers where pathologists specializing in rare tumors could examine the samples: Mayo Clinic in Rochester, Minnesota; M. D. Anderson Medical Center in Houston; and Air Force Pathology in Washington, D.C., were just a few.

For a second time in a little over a year I was told to wait. I had hoped the results of this biopsy would solve the mystery so I could either put this all behind me or get on to dealing with the problem. Instead I was in limbo again. One day I would feel the ordeal was nearly over; the next day I would wonder if I was going to die before I graduated from high school.

During this waiting period, God let me meet many people who had handicaps or limitations. I talked with them and watched how they dealt with their disability and suffering. I sensed a special bond with them and felt God had intentionally arranged for our paths to cross.

## The Fateful Phone Call

A month went by after my second biopsy. Then Christmas came and went. January and February passed. March was nearly half over. Dr. Kline was receiving mixed professional opinions about the tumor samples. Some pathologists concluded it was a benign lesion, while others said it was a malignant tumor. Still others continued to be baffled. Dr. Kline called us as reports came in.

Our family was assuming from the initial reports that I probably would have a bone replacement. We expected Dr. Kline to call at any time to let us know the best date for me to go to Houston for surgery.

We didn't know at the time how much he agonized, weighing all the pros and cons. Finally, with the counsel of many experts, he reluctantly decided on what he felt was the most medically sound course of action.

I remember the evening Dr. Kline called. I answered the phone and recognized his voice. I expected him to say, "Well, Becki, you need to go to Houston on such-and-such a date." Instead he wanted to talk to my dad. I heard Dad say, "No, I'm sorry we can't get together for a consultation tonight. We have to attend the annual congregational meeting at the church."

Dr. Kline gently insisted that he needed to talk to my parents right away and said he would meet them at church. A part of me sensed something was very wrong; otherwise Dr. Kline would have given me the information, since I had a very open relationship with him.

My parents left for the meeting, and I continued watering plants and baking brownies. Our whole family was leaving soon for a spring vacation in Florida, and I was getting ready for our trip.

**The Doctor's House Call**
Suddenly my parents came home—long before the meeting was scheduled to end. Mom and Dad had met with Dr. Kline before the meeting. They felt it was more important to come back home to talk to me than attend the meeting. I knew right away that they had bad news. Their faces were very serious, and their eyes were red. A huge cloud of gloom came through the door with them.

Dr. Kline followed Mom and Dad into the house. Now I was certain that something was very wrong! Dr. Kline had a somber look on his face and said, "We need to talk." We all went into the living room to sit down. He carefully explained that the biopsy results had convinced him that the tumor was potentially dangerous to my life. He said, "I wish there were another way, but the only answer is—amputation."

## Knowing—Finally

It was strange, but at the moment Dr. Kline explained the need for an amputation, I had a number of feelings—shock, excitement, curiosity and peace. Even though I was shocked, I had been having an underlying suspicion that it was coming, so the news wasn't totally unexpected. In many ways, I felt that God was starting me on an exciting adventure.

I didn't feel angry. In fact, I was relieved to finally know exactly what was wrong. I also felt responsible to help my parents. They seemed totally destroyed by this news. I wanted to show them that I'd make it through this.

Although the tumor had not been easily diagnosed, several national experts on rare tumors had decided this growth was an unusual type of cancer that would grow rather slowly for a number of years. In fact, it may have been there for a long time. These doctors believed that one day it would enlarge enough to break out of the bone wall, thus having the potential to spread to other areas of my body.[1] This diagnosis had caused Dr. Kline to conclude that something drastic had to be done. During the past months he had been consulting with doctors all over the United States about various possible procedures. One suggestion was to replace part of my leg bone by removing the affected section of my femur and putting in a prosthetic (false bone) portion. Another was to graft in a new section of human bone. Still another procedure was amputation.

The problem with having the bone replaced was that I'd have to be on medication to keep my body from rejecting the foreign matter. This medication would make it impossible to use chemotherapy to eradicate the cancer. Research showed a poorer prognosis in patients who had bone replacements because the cancer could spread, fatally attacking their lungs or other organs. It was also more likely that the cancer would spread at the surgical site with this method than with an amputation.

I was very curious about what to expect now that the amputation was a necessity. I asked a lot of questions about the artificial leg I would have. Dr. Kline told me the prosthetist in our city was an extraordinary craftsman who could make a very natural-looking leg.

I also had a more immediate question: Could our family still go to Florida for spring break? Even though Dr. Kline wanted to do the surgery right away, without too much pressure I talked him into letting us go on our vacation. I convinced him that it would be important for my psychological well-being! After the long, dreary Illinois winter, I was counting on getting a suntan.

## An Exciting Adventure

More than anything else, I felt a deep responsibility to God. I was excited because I sensed God was going to use me in special ways. I wanted to serve him and not disappoint him. I felt God was giving me a big opportunity, and I didn't want to lose it by being selfish or self-absorbed.

Weeks before, I had been asking God where he wanted me to go to college and what profession he wanted me to pursue. Now I felt that God was clearly answering my prayer—maybe not in the way I thought he would, but in a distinct way all the same. It was as if he were saying, "I have a specific mission for you, and I need to change you so that you'll fit in with what I have planned."

God could have used my life if I had two legs, but I'm not

sure I would have been as open to his plans. I was easily distracted by my strengths and abilities. When the need for my amputation came, I saw this as God's way of tailoring me for a specific service—one I might not have been able to do as well with a whole, healthy body. I now would be able to understand loss in other people's lives. Because I sensed the surgery was God's direct will, the transition to being an amputee was easier. Why should I feel angry when God was accomplishing his plan for me?

In those minutes with Dr. Kline in our living room, I thought to myself, "I don't want to miss the opportunity God is giving me." I was excited that he was working so definitely in my life. I hadn't always responded that way to circumstances. But in this situation I felt very strongly that the Holy Spirit was doing fantastic things in me and would use me in an unusual way.

My faith didn't just begin that night. I had been committed to God for many years, and it came naturally for me to trust God with something this big. I knew I didn't have answers in myself; I had to trust God. From my earliest years, I had learned at home and in church about God's love and that he had plans for my life. As a young child, I had taken responsibility for my decision to accept Christ and my walk with God.

When I was only four years old, I was attracted to Jesus because of his forgiveness. From my view of life, I needed it quite often! I wasn't a bad kid, but I did have the typical poor judgment of a pre-schooler. Due to my boundless energy, I often acted before I thought through the consequences. As a result, I found myself being disciplined on a regular basis. My limited understanding of God was that he loved me regardless of my mistakes and he would always forgive me. My mom tells me I had a very tender conscience, and I frequently came to her for help in asking for God's pardon.

## The Ruse

I remember one time in particular when God's forgiveness was very powerful. I was barely seven when, during my bath one evening, we discovered a lump on my abdomen. It was diagnosed as a hernia by my pediatrician, and a few days later I had surgery.

During my recovery I received a humorous get well card that included punch-out glasses and a mustache to use as a disguise to sneak out of the hospital. When my parents came to visit, I told them that I had put on the disguise and was halfway down the hall before a nurse barked, "What are you doing out of bed without your slippers?"

I was adventuresome enough to have actually tried a stunt like that, so my story was believable. But it was fabricated. I had been scolded for being in the hall without my slippers, but I had never tried the "get away getup."

It wouldn't have been so bad if the lie had stopped there, but it spread. Thinking it was such a cute story, Mom and Dad shared the antic with several friends. I squirmed every time I heard them repeat it.

Finally, one night as I lay in bed, I heard my unsuspecting mom reciting my big lie on the phone to yet another person. I felt awful. I began to cry. How could I have deceived so many people?

I called Mom to my room. Through my tears I told her the truth and that I was very sorry for lying. We prayed together for my forgiveness, and I felt a tremendous burden lift from my heart. Jesus was very personal and close to me.

My growing trust in God continued as I assumed more responsibility for my life. When I was about twelve, I began to spend time alone praying and reading my Bible. It wasn't something anyone told me to do. I had seen a daily quiet time modeled by my mom. Every morning when I got up, I found her sitting in the living room praying. Often our family cat would be sharing her lap with her Bible.

Part of my quiet time at age twelve involved keeping a journal. One section was for prayer requests and God's answers. Through this simple form of documentation, I clearly saw God at work in my life. I began to trust his guidance in bigger and more important areas. By the time I reached my teen years, I was accustomed to trusting God for his best in my life.

## Using My Whole Body

After Dr. Kline left that night, I convinced my parents to go back to their church meeting. I knew I needed to tell someone, so I phoned my best friend, Raewyn, and asked her if she could come over. She had been following developments all along and was expecting that I would have the bone-replacement operation.

When she arrived, I gave her the news. After I explained that the doctor said I would be having my leg removed, we sat down on a bed and prayed. I don't remember exactly what we prayed about, but again I felt a deep sense that God was working in me and was in control. Both of us experienced an incredible peace that God had a reason for this event. Raewyn didn't need to say anything profound to me. It was enough to have her with me.

Then we did something fun. We realized I had only a short time left with two legs. With the surgery scheduled in two weeks, I wanted to get the most I could out of those days. I decided to enjoy all my body while I had it. Raewyn helped me move the living room furniture out of the way. Then we put on some records, and—as I had done so often for many years—we exhausted ourselves doing gymnastics across the living room floor for more than an hour.

Fully enjoying my two-leggedness became my goal for our

family vacation in Florida. I was a junior in high school and in the middle of track season, so I was in good physical shape. In Florida I spent a lot of time running on the beach and enjoying the whole body God had given me. I was glad I had those extra days to run and jump. I often looked at my leg and sort of said good-by to it.

I also enjoyed my two good legs when we were driving back from Florida. We had been cooped up in our borrowed motor home for several hours and needed to stretch. At a rest area in Georgia, we all jumped out and started running around. I sprinted my hardest from the bathroom back to the motor home.

It was wonderful to throw my whole body into running as hard as I could. I loved feeling strong and healthy. I enjoyed the feeling of my heart beating, arms and legs pumping, and everything working in harmony. How exhilarating it was to run.

"What a great gift our bodies are!" I thought. "Maybe this is going to be one of the last times I get to sprint like this—until I'm in heaven and have a new body."

## A Transition Time

The restful time in Florida was important for my family and me to adjust to my impending operation. We spent a lot of time talking. My sister, Barbara, who was at the University of Illinois that semester and living at home, already knew about the coming amputation. But we still had to break the news to my other sister, Brenda. She was a student at Taylor University and had already left for Florida when we learned I would have surgery. I remember how hard it was to tell her when we finally all met in Florida.

It felt good for our whole family to be together. The Cox family, our close friends, along with Raewyn and Barbara's former roommate, joined in this special time. We were serious, but we joked a lot too. I thought of all kinds of weird things, such as what I was going to do with my extra pant leg. Obviously, I couldn't just have it blowing around in the wind. Everyone came up with ideas. I finally suggested sewing a brick in the bottom of the pant leg.

I tried to imagine what it would be like to walk with a fake leg. One time when I was walking from the camper to the restroom, I tried limping as I thought I would with a prothesis. Now I realize I had the movements all wrong. I don't really drag my artificial leg like the hunchback of Notre Dame.

The discussions and jokes helped prepare all of us. We also spent time praying that God would miraculously heal me. We knew that God was bigger than any illness. If it were his will, he could remove the tumor. But we also prayed that he would meet our needs, no matter what his plan was for my leg.

I really felt my parents' grief during those days. At times I saw them looking at me with a deep sadness. I heard them talking in the back bedroom of the camper, and I could sense their pain by the tone of their voices. They felt out of control and couldn't do anything about what was going to happen to me. They loved and supported me, but they couldn't take away the cancer. Many times they told me that if it were possible, they'd be glad to give one of their legs in my place. They didn't like feeling helpless and not able to "make it all better."

## Would God Heal?

We got home from Florida on Sunday. The next day I was admitted to the hospital and given all the routine tests. That evening my family gathered around my hospital bed to pray again for God to heal me. I had been anointed by the church elders earlier, and people were praying around the clock, asking God for my healing.

As we prayed in my hospital room that evening, I felt the

tension between what I thought was inevitable and what my father believed would happen. Dad was confident that I would be healed.

During the days prior to surgery Dad had asked, "Do you feel God is going to heal you?" I responded, "I know God *can* heal, but I'm not sure it's his will at this time." Saying that to my dad was really difficult because he so much wanted my healing to be God's will.

I'd seen other people healed; yet, somehow, I just didn't sense it was going to happen to me. God had prepared me for the worst. In some ways, it would have been anticlimactic for him to heal me. It seemed as if he'd been preparing me for something much more than a healing. I felt that God was going to change my whole life.

Perhaps I wouldn't have been thankful for the healing very long. When God answers my prayers, I thank him and then usually forget about it. If God had healed me, a few weeks later I might have been back in my old routine. I would have been thankful at the time, but the ordeal would have been over and forgotten—except as a great story for a Bible study meeting.

If I had told my non-Christian friends I'd been healed, they would have said, "Sure, Becki, we always knew you were a little strange." It would have been hard for them to believe a healing had taken place inside my sturdy, tanned leg that looked healthy on the outside.

The next morning, as I was being wheeled on the gurney from my hospital room to surgery, my dad walked alongside, holding my hand. At the elevator before he, Mom and my sisters had to say good-by to me, Dad said, "Don't worry, Honey, you're going to be back in just a little while. They're going to open up your leg and find that the cancer's gone."

I wanted to believe that for his sake, but I honestly didn't feel healing was God's plan for me. Instead I felt God's incredible

strength and sensed tremendous courage that I'd never possessed previously. I'd never had to trust God for something this
big before, but I felt wonderfully buoyed up by his power. I was
sure God was in control and present with me every second.

## Farewell

As I went to the operating room, I was completely alert. I had
requested not to have the pre-op medication given to make a
patient drowsy before surgery. Those shots always made me
sick, so I preferred not to have one. I talked and joked with the
nurses and orderlies who were attending me on the way to the
operating room. I was keenly aware of the seriousness of what
was going to happen in the next few minutes, but I felt relaxed
and secure in God's love.

As I waited on the gurney while it was stopped outside the
operating room, I was able to look out a window. It was a
beautiful spring day with a crystal blue sky. I thought, "To
anybody else, this is just a normal Tuesday. To me, this day is
going to change the rest of my life."

When I was wheeled into the operating room, I saw the big
instrument they would use to take off my leg. I was very curious about all that was going to happen and asked questions
until they gave me the anesthetic. I was not afraid, because I
felt God was right there holding my hand, assuring me that he
was in control and would use this to his glory.

Earlier that morning the nurses had asked me to "prep" the
surgical area of my body. I shaved my entire leg and scrubbed
it with Benedyne for fifteen minutes to make sure it was sterile.
I looked at how tan that leg had become in Florida. How athletic and healthy it looked from the outside! I thanked God for
all he had given me, and then I said "good-by" to my left leg.

# 3

## A MOTHER'S PERSPECTIVE

# I HELPED
# MAKE THAT LEG

**D**r. Kline, Jim and I were sitting in a tight little circle on cold, metal folding chairs in a dimly lit church room. That March evening in 1978 Dr. Kline was explaining the latest conclusions regarding Becki's tumor. The surroundings were unfamiliar to me because we were borrowing another church for our congregational dinner-meeting that night. The building was bustling with activity, but we had found a quiet space behind a sliding partition in a large room. The area seemed dark and cold, but perhaps that was only because I was feeling apprehensive.

When I fully realized that Dr. Kline was saying Becki would need her left leg removed, I was stunned. I thought, "What a waste of a good leg. Why, I helped *make* that leg!"

## God's Third Gift

I began to reminisce about my pregnancy with Becki. We were so glad to be having our third baby. We had carefully considered whether we should have any more children because of Nikita Khruschev's flagrant boast that our nation would be under Communist rule by 1970. We didn't want any of our children to be too young to have made a personal commitment to the Lord if our freedom of religion would be taken from us.

However, in early 1961 we decided we needed at least one more child to round out our family, which already included two daughters, Barbara and Brenda. We vowed to do our human part in seeing our children come to Christ at an early age.

We had learned that conception took place under irregular circumstances for us, so we were delighted when I was pregnant again. We appreciated what a special miracle was taking place inside me as God carefully formed this third baby. Of course, we assumed God was making this one to be a boy!

Jim and I were together in the delivery room on September 27, 1961. (In those days fathers had to have special permission to be present at a birth.) As the baby's head emerged, the obstetrician looked up at Jim and asked, "Well, what do you want? A boy or a girl?" Jim nervously exclaimed, "Never mind that. Just get on with the delivery!" In minutes we were both falling in love with our third darling girl and named her Becky Kay. (Becki was spelled with a *y* until age fifteen when she decided to change it.)

As she grew in the first months after birth, she had an extra little roll of baby fat near the top of one of her legs. A family friend lovingly called it "Becky's little sausage roll." By the time she was sixteen, of course, Becki made sure she had no fat rolls anywhere. I no longer could remember which leg had had the cute little sausage roll, but I wondered if that was the one to be cut off.

## When It Rains It Pours

In the dark shadows of the church room that dreary March night, I started to cry. It was the first time I had cried during the whole ordeal that had begun a year and a half before. Dr. Kline said sympathetically, "That's O.K., Sally. You've been so strong through everything. It's O.K. to cry."

By "everything," he was referring to all that had hit our family in the previous months. In addition to Becki's two major biopsy surgeries, he had seen Jim—his pastor—struggle with a severe case of mononucleosis and a traumatic mid-life crisis. He had been treating our oldest daughter, Barbara, for a complicated broken collarbone that had not healed in five months (and didn't heal for another year). Earlier he had cared for Brenda's broken foot. We also had recently had two other cases of mono, injuries from two car accidents, Brenda's severe viral infection and head concussion, and a list of other illnesses and injuries.

While we were being heavily besieged with the family's physical problems and Jim's mid-life stress that previous November, a friend asked, "Wow! What is God doing to the Conways?"

I blithely answered, "Oh, I guess he's just getting us ready for something bigger."

My philosophy had always been that trials in our lives are used by the Lord to strengthen us for the next test. That test might be harder, but it wouldn't be impossible because he had been preparing us.

*33*

## Heavy Darkness

Those words to my friend came shouting back through the circuits of my mind the following January as Becki and I saw Dr. Kline for a follow-up visit after her second biopsy. For the first time, he had received some negative reports about her tumor samples.

At earlier post-operative visits, he had reported that the various pathologists around the nation weren't sure what type of tumor it was, but it seemed to be benign. We had begun to assume that all was well. Now those hopes were being splintered.

I felt as if I had lead pellets in the bottom of my stomach as we walked out of the medical clinic into the black, winter night. It had been daylight when we entered, but night had come quickly in more than one way. Echoing through my brain paths were those words, "Oh, I guess he's just getting us ready for something bigger."

How would I tell Jim? He had just begun to recover somewhat from his serious mid-life depression. For over two years my emotionally and spiritually strong husband had been struggling to survive. Instead of his usual optimism, he had not been able to see anything right with the world. He was at the point of running away to escape his misery when God renewed him with hope that he would eventually recover. He was out of the pit for longer periods of time now, but I also knew that it didn't take much to put him back into despair.[1]

Of course, I *would* tell him about Becki's ominous report. We had always shared everything about the family and drawn strength from each other. Together we had relied on the Lord who had brought us through many problems in the past and surely would again. Yet I dreaded telling him this bad news when he wasn't as strong as usual.

Jim didn't say much when I told him Dr. Kline's news. He seemed to take his pre-mid-life-crisis attitude toward uncertain situations: "Let's not get excited one way or the other until all the facts are in." He was certain God would intervene.

I could feel myself bracing for whatever would be "something bigger." I wasn't scared; I just wanted to be able to help everyone through this time. I knew that God's plan was always one of love.

## Winning in the Hard Times

My assurance of God's good purposes came from many times in the past when God had done what was best for me despite difficult circumstances. Ever since I had made a definite commitment of my life to Christ as a college freshman, I had experienced the Lord's care for me and, later, for our family.

Actually, my foundation for trusting in God's love began when I was born to a mother and father who loved me and made me feel very valued. I always knew they were on my side when I had a problem or was facing the challenge of learning something new.

When I was sick or injured, they made it easy to get well by giving me the extra care I needed. Many times they wrapped and unwrapped cloth bandages from the many injuries I received while growing up! (My childhood was in the days before Band-Aids.) Mother was a tender nurse. She would bring special foods on a cookie sheet disguised as a bed tray and help me entertain myself until I was well again. My parents' attention to my needs taught me that God would meet my needs.

Mother and Daddy were good examples of how a family cares for each other and makes it through tough times. We were farmers, and my brother and I were born just after the Great Depression. Of course, Tommy and I didn't even realize our economic difficulties as we grew up. What we did see was Mother and Daddy's love for each other and for us as they faced crop failures, price drops, hailstorms, droughts, livestock deaths and our own personal illnesses.

## What Really Counts

One evening after a summer storm, Mother stood beside me outside our house. We leaned on the rain-dampened fence that separated our little yard of grass and flowers from the rest of the farmyard. We were looking across a small valley to the next hill where our corn crop had just been shredded by hail. The friendly evening sun was lighting the sky after the heavy green storm clouds had angrily rolled on to continue dumping their destructive load of hail on other farmers' fields. The air now smelled clean. But a big portion of our year's income lay pounded into a sickening mass on the ground over on that hill.

I knew Mother grieved over the work and expense that had gone into that cornfield. She probably said something about all that, but what I remember is her arm around my shoulder and her words, "You know, Honey, a husband and wife can take anything that comes in life as long as they love each other."

## Recounting the Past

After telling Jim about the negative reports on Becki's tumor that January night, I lay awake a long time. Silently I rehearsed the events since we had learned over a year earlier that her knee trouble was more than growing pains and normal bruises.

I was grateful that the doctor correcting Becki's displaced tailbone had insisted on x-raying her knee the day she limped into his office. I wondered why our pediatrician and the first orthopedist hadn't taken x-rays. I somewhat convinced myself that they were not to be blamed since they each felt it was a temporary condition. But I couldn't help but wonder if the prognosis now would be more hopeful if they had detected the tumor during one of those early visits.

I was thankful that Dr. Kline was now on the orthopedic staff at the clinic and was using the nation's best resources to study Becki's tumor. I appreciated his warm-hearted honesty. I knew he cared for us, and I trusted his professional skills.

I thought of how my emotions had risen and fallen since we first learned of Becki's tumor. At the time of her first biopsy, I had been scared of "the worst"—deadly cancer spreading throughout her body. Then, when the reports seemed to be hopeful, my spirits soared. All we had to do was help Becki recover from the drastic incision in her upper leg muscle. Then came the need for a second biopsy. The initial reports were optimistic. So were my feelings. Now, with reports of a cancer possibility, my emotions were dipping again.

## Growing Up Quickly

In spite of threats of impending problems, I couldn't forget the good things that were happening. I was pleased that Becki was flowering spiritually and God was very personal to her. One day as she and I drove to the clinic for another round of tests before the first biopsy, she talked about some insights she had from her daily quiet times.

She was especially impressed with 2 Corinthians 4:16-17: "Though our bodies are dying, our inner strength in the Lord is growing every day. These troubles and sufferings of ours are, after all, quite small and won't last very long. Yet this short time of distress will result in God's richest blessing upon us forever and ever!" (LB).

"So, Mom," she had said, "even though we don't know what all this is going to bring, it's only for the short time I am here on earth, and that's nothing compared to the good things I'll enjoy forever in heaven."

I was proud of her maturity. Even after the first biopsy reports had come back as "probably benign" and we felt safe again, she had a sharpened focus on what was truly important in life. Sure, she still made some typically fifteen-year-old choices and had the normal adolescent ups-and-downs during that year after the first biopsy. But overall God was sculpting a significant work. She had a clear perspective on eternal values rather than on appearance or popularity. She was sensitive to other people with problems and also was determined to live her life as normally as possible.

I admired her hard work to get back in shape for the track team. She started in late winter by using an indoor track while it was too cold to run outdoors. That left leg had a lot of recovering to do to get ready for hurdles again.

As the track season started, she wasn't quite as good as she had been the year before. I was irritated with the coaches who only criticized her and didn't give her credit for what she was overcoming. I wanted to say, "Listen here! You should be patting her on the back for how well she's doing." (Of course, that was just a little motherly prejudice.)

I chuckled as I thought of Becki's nickname around the medical clinic. We heard about it one day as a white-coated doctor got on the elevator in which we were riding. Becki was still on crutches following the first surgery. She and I were engrossed in a conversation in which I called her by name. The doctor looked at her and said, "Becki? You must be Becki Conway, the Mystery Girl."

Becki said, "Yes, I'm Becki Conway, but. . . ."

"Well, everyone around here calls you the Mystery Girl because your tumor is such a mystery to us. We can't figure out what it is. By the way, I'm one of the pathologists here."

## A Timely Gift

I continued to reminisce before I went to sleep that January night. I smiled as I thought how God had providentially arranged for our local Christian bookstore manager to give us a complimentary copy of the new book, *Joni,* about the time we discovered Becki's tumor. He didn't even know about our need, but God did.

I carried the book with me as Becki and I went to her various medical appointments. I read part of it while waiting for her to have her first CAT scan. That procedure was relatively new at the time. I was struggling with having my daughter injected with radioactive material and being moved through some strange machine behind closed doors I wasn't allowed to enter. All I could do was wait in the hall. I was glad to have the book to read.

As Becki and I went from department to department in the clinic, I shared what I had just read from Joni's story. Then I'd read some more while I waited for Becki to go through the next test.

Imagine our delight when we learned that Joni was coming to Urbana. She was to speak at a mother–daughter breakfast and then hold a citywide meeting in our church.

Becki was out of the hospital, with her deep leg wound still healing from the biopsy, when Joni came. I was so proud to attend the breakfast with Becki beside me on her crutches. That evening we went with Jim to Joni's meeting at our church.

We had been profoundly affected by Joni's life through her book, but hearing her in person made an even deeper impression on us. Her message was powerful as she deftly illustrated her points by creating a picture with a pen in her mouth. We were watching God's grace at work: Joni's seeming tragedy being used in triumph for many other people's lives.

As I lay recalling past events that January night, I realized how good God's timing was to allow Joni's life to touch ours when it did. We were to cross paths with her many times in the years to follow, but I didn't know that then.

**Short Return to Normalcy**

With the optimistic reports from the first biopsy and her leg muscle and incision healed, Becki's life began to be normal once more. That summer she climbed Horn Peak, a 13,000-foot Colorado mountain. But in the fall she began to limp again. After more x-rays and tests, Dr. Kline scheduled the second biopsy. In the light of her past history of injuries and operations, I thought the surgery date was appropriate—Veteran's Day!

Becki's surgery on Veteran's Day came a few days after I made an urgent trip to Taylor University where both of our other daughters had been hospitalized. Brenda had been admitted to the student health center with a serious viral infection. Then Barbara had had a bike accident and sustained a compound fracture of her collarbone. She couldn't use either arm and was in great pain.

When I arrived at the health center late that night, I found Barbara in one bed, but Brenda's bed was empty. She had been taken to another hospital to be x-rayed for a head concussion. When she had heard that Barbara was hurt and in the next room, she hurriedly jumped out of bed to comfort Barbara. In her weakened condition, she fainted and hit her head as she fell.

I stayed a few days, helping care for both girls, and eventually brought Barbara home for more care. Jim was already home, taking a month's leave of absence from his pastoral duties to try to regain his stability from his mid-life crisis. On top of everything, we were facing the unknown about Becki's tumor again. Veteran's Day was very significant for all of us.

**Thanks-giving**

Becki had a heavy cast on her leg as she recovered from her second biopsy. By this time we were into the holiday season. We had a wonderful reason to celebrate on Thanksgiving Day, because it was during the night before that God had showed Jim in a very special way that he was going to make it through the dreadful confusion of his mid-life crisis.[2] Before our Thanksgiving dinner he read to us from Psalm 18, which God had led him to read as he awoke that morning. We all rejoiced that the Lord had "reached down from heaven" and drawn Jim "out of (his) great trials."

## Another Scare

Mixed with Christmas and a few rounds of flu for everyone was the dilemma of how to meet the publisher's January 15 deadline for Jim's first book, *Men in Mid-Life Crisis.* Jim had nearly given up on it, but with his restored fervor he decided that we could do it if we both worked day and night. We started pushing hard to get it done.

Now, ten days before the deadline, we had received these disappointing reports about Becki's tumor when she and I had seen Dr. Kline at the clinic that dark evening. Time to stop reminiscing and get to sleep, if I were to keep up with everything!

Miraculously, we finished the book manuscript. But in the very last weary hours of typing the final pages, Becki came to me with a concerned look on her face. "Mom," she said hesitantly, not wanting to interrupt my work on the book, "I've just found a big lump in my breast."

She didn't know if it were anything to be troubled about, but it was very painful. "Oh, no!" I thought. "She *does* have cancer, and it is spreading to the other parts of her body!"

My mind was in a whirl. I wanted to call Dr. Kline right away, but it was the weekend and I hated to interrupt him at home. We decided I should call anyway. He graciously listened to me. Then he assured me that—although we were justifiably concerned about cancer—the lump probably was benign, especially since it was painful and had appeared suddenly. Tests in the next few days proved him to be correct.

## Wrestling Alone

During the rest of January we continued to wait for more reports on the bone tumor, hoping the next ones would overrule the bad ones. They didn't. Dr. Kline began to talk about our next steps. He and the other specialists were thinking that perhaps the best procedure would be to send Becki to M. D. Anderson Medical Center in Houston.

In the meantime, I went with Jim on a long-planned trip to California for two weeks. I audited classes with him as he worked on his Doctor of Ministry degree at Fuller Theological Seminary. In between classes we enjoyed the warmth and beauty of California, feeling smug that we were escaping the snowstorms of Illinois.

When we were in our hotel room one evening, Becki telephoned. She was home alone that night and was going through a difficult time. After school she had received a call from someone at the medical clinic who talked at length about the reports from her second biopsy and what her prognosis was. The person told her she would probably go to Houston to have that section of her bone removed and other bone grafted into that area. The realization of what this actually meant was very unsettling to Becki as she struggled alone that evening. We were bothered, too, and felt sad that we couldn't be with her in her time of suffering.

## Waiting—Waiting

The days following those first traumatic reports stretched into weeks, and we heard very little about what the doctors were deciding. The last word was about the bone graft, so I made preliminary plans for transportation to Houston and housing near the hospital, but nothing definite could be arranged.

Sometimes my thoughts turned to life *after* the operation. Dr. Kline had told us she would have to wear a metal leg brace for two or three years while the bone graft became a complete part of her leg. I thought, "Oh, dear, that means she'll go off to college looking like a cripple. People won't know that she hasn't always been that way." That would be embarrassing, yet I would certainly be able to accept it if it meant saving Becki's life.

Four months passed after her second biopsy, and my impatience was growing because we hadn't heard more definite details about going to Houston. "On the other hand," I thought, "perhaps this is a good sign. If they're in no hurry, maybe it means she won't have to have anything done."

## The End of the Waiting

Then came that telephone call from Dr. Kline the evening of March 14. "Can you meet me right away for a consultation about Becki's tumor?" he asked.

We reminded him that this was the night of our annual church meeting. Some unusually urgent matters were to be discussed, and Jim had prepared an important and complicated presentation that only he could give. We felt we had to be at that meeting. We arranged to meet Dr. Kline at the church before the meeting, not realizing the gravity of what he had to say.

After talking to Jim and me at the church, Dr. Kline followed us to the house to share the bad news with Becki. I was amazed at her acceptance and sense of humor. I personally was still in shock. When Becki encouraged Jim and me to go back to our church meeting, I went, feeling stoic and courageous. Probably I was just numb.

We joined the meeting in progress and Jim made his presentation. He didn't reveal the news that we'd just learned Becki needed the amputation. The business meeting continued, and I began to feel agitated with people who seemed to have petty attitudes about matters that seemed so insignificant. I was sitting there struggling with a new perspective on the real issues of life.

I usually didn't speak up much at church business meetings, but suddenly I found myself openly disputing with a young man over whether or not to spend money to send some staff out of state for evangelism training. I realized later that my anger was misplaced. I should not even have been in a meeting like that while dealing with the fresh blow about Becki.

## The Countdown

We left for Florida soon after the news. The vacation was filled with bittersweet days—sweet to be together as a family; bitter to know we were coming home to Becki's amputation. That was a cherished time, however, and very important for our preparation. In addition to the two girlfriends of our daughters, our very special friends, the Coxes, were with us. Their love and concern were also part of God's provision.

The day after we arrived home from Florida, I helped Becki get admitted to the hospital. Then I went to the grocery store. As I pulled into a parking space and saw people coming and going from the store where I had been shopping for nearly nine years, I thought, "No one even knows that I am the mother of a girl about to get her leg cut off."

I entered the store and picked up my groceries. I was in a familiar place, carrying out a familiar task, but I felt very strange and alone. The check-out clerks who had waited on me for years didn't know something so drastic was about to happen in my life. Somehow I thought my new circumstances ought to be emblazoned on me for all to see.

Jim and some of our friends had been more certain than I that God would perform a last-minute miracle and heal Becki's leg. I had been praying fervently, too, but I wasn't as confident.

In one of our chats, Becki had acknowledged to me, "I know that God has the ability to heal me, but I'm not sure he is going to."

I nodded and said, "I know he can, and I want him to heal you, but I also don't have the peace that he is going to."

Early on the morning of March 28, 1978, Jim and I prepared to go to the hospital to be with Becki before she was taken to surgery. The atmosphere in our bedroom was strange. Part of me was at perfect peace, knowing that God was totally in control of whatever was to happen. Another part of me felt a mixture of hope and dread, wondering whether or not God was going to remove that tumor before surgery.

Jim was sitting dejectedly on the bed, not moving to get dressed. Finally, he shook his head and said, "What do you wear on the day your daughter is supposed to get her leg chopped off?"

The four of us—Jim, Barbara, Brenda and I—were at the hospital in time to be with Becki for several minutes before surgery. We had come to encourage her, but instead her courage and wit were a strength to us. We prayed with her and committed her to God's care.

She was wheeled off to surgery as she chatted and joked with the attendants. She left with the two legs I had "helped make." Would she return with one or both?

We went to the waiting room where a huge crowd of friends was gathering to be with us. My body sat down in a comfortable chair, but my heart and mind were in that operating room.

# 4

## A FATHER'S PERSPECTIVE

# GOD WILL WORK A MIRACLE

*At the time Becki's tumor was discovered, I was pastor* of Twin City Bible Church in Urbana, Illinois. This was a church that believed God heard and answered prayer, and nothing was too hard for him.

Our congregation of approximately 1500 people had a well-structured care-group program. The church was mostly made up of University of Illinois students, many of whom belonged to various small groups. In addition, dozens of non-student groups were organized under one of our pastors. We also had developed several prayer chains in the church so that prayer needs could be shared quickly.

When Becki's tumor was discovered, we were glad for the efficient network of prayer support. It helped us to know that people in the prayer chains, small groups and Sunday-school classes were praying for Becki and our family as we went through her first biopsy.

A corporate sigh of relief arose when the first biopsy reports revealed that the growth in Becki's leg was not malignant. The doctors warned that it was a mysterious tumor, however, and needed to be watched.

## Second Biopsy

When Becki entered the hospital for her second biopsy, the church was once more mobilized for prayer. Again we received hundreds of verbal and written assurances that people were daily asking God for his healing in Becki's life.

After the second biopsy, the pathologists' reports came back with mixed opinions. Some specialists thought the tumor was malignant while others did not. However, the consensus was that, whether malignant or not, the tumor should be removed because it was continuing to grow. Unknown to us, the discussion among the specialists around the nation now centered on whether to remove just the affected area and replace it with a bone transplant or to remove the entire leg.

The deliberations of what to do went on from November into March of the following year with very little information coming to us. People continued to pray, but because we were not hearing regular updates on the progress of the decision from the specialists, the intensity of prayer began to wane.

## A Grim Night

On that fateful March evening, Dr. Scott Kline called our house to let us know that he wanted to talk to us. My reactions to his call and subsequent visit were very different from Becki's.

Scott was a member of our church, a personal friend and in charge of the decision about Becki's leg. As we all seated ourselves in the living room for him to talk to us, the atmosphere seemed heavy and depressive to me. Scott sat on the edge of his chair and told us that the opinions were all in. Becki had a slow-growing, malignant tumor that needed to be removed.

He explained the options, with the advantages and disadvantages of each, and then said, "The best of all the solutions is that the leg be removed so that the cancer cannot spread. Because the tumor has affected the upper part of the knee joint, it would be impossible to do a bone graft and still have a workable knee. Amputation is the only answer."

I asked, "What about chemotherapy or radiation?" He said the growth was too massive and neither of these procedures would be effective. He followed it up by saying that he wanted to have Becki admitted for surgery as soon as possible.

It was a grim moment. What do you say when you've just been told that your sixteen-year-old daughter is going to have her left leg cut off more than halfway up her thigh? How could anyone have the courage to take the scalpel and saw in hand and cut through that strong, young, muscular leg that had so recently been running track, climbing our backyard tree fort, bicycling, swimming and doing the Chinese splits as a cheerleader?

I sat there in numbed silence. But Becki, with her unusual wit and her deep commitment to God, rescued me. Scott had just finished explaining about the prosthesis she would have. She was thinking about the Florida suntan she hoped to get and how the prosthetist would provide a natural-looking leg if she were sometimes tan. She asked Dr. Kline, "Well, am I going to have a summer leg and a winter leg? A dark one to match my summer tan and a light one for wintertime?"

I was shocked by what seemed to be her totally inappropri-ate question to the doctor. How could she joke about this? What made her seem to brush it off so coolly? Her ability to express humor and to see God in the process yanked me up out of the pit. I began to get perspective, to gain hope and to again believe God was going to do something great!

## The College Years of Faith

Our family has always had a deep consciousness of God's work in the world and in our personal lives. Sally and I both became Christians at the beginning of our college years and expe-rienced hundreds of answers to prayer. God provided small things like meal tickets, as well as unexpected money for our tuition and books. God's calling me into full-time ministry was an act of his special work as he developed my faith.

While I was a freshman at Sterling College in central Kansas, I met each day with a small group of college guys who were very significant to my spiritual growth. We prayed for each other, asking for God's guidance and provision for our lives. God caused us to grow rapidly and gave us capacities and opportunities beyond our native abilities. We watched him use our ordinary lives to make a spiritual difference on the campus and as we preached and sang in jails, retirement homes, other colleges and churches. We saw people place their faith in Jesus Christ or recommit themselves to a deeper walk with Jesus.

On one occasion our team was making a return visit to a jail where we had ministered about six months earlier. Several of the men seemed extremely hard and withdrawn as we were ushered into the cell block. I was surprised to see a chalk drawing depicting the resurrection of Jesus Christ taped on a wall inside one of the cells. I recognized the picture as one I had drawn during my first visit to this jail when I shared the good news of Christ's personal forgiveness.

Innocently, I said I liked the picture on the wall and asked who had drawn it. Three men from the back of the group pushed their way to the front. They said they didn't know who had drawn the picture, but it had been given to another inmate who had since been transferred to a different prison. That inmate had become a Christian when that picture was drawn and had in turn led these three men to Christ. The first man had started a Bible study with them. The men said this picture had become a symbol to them that God really loved them.

Standing right before my eyes were three of my spiritual grandsons! God *was* doing miracles, and he was allowing me to share in that process.

### Answers Continue

God gave me the privilege of being a student pastor of two small churches during my junior and senior years of college. In one church, eleven of twelve kids in the youth group came to a personal relationship with Christ during my time with them.

After Sally and I were married, the process of God's good work in us continued. We prayed about everything. Our prayers were answered as God formed our character and directed our ministry with people.

We spent three years in Denver, where I attended seminary. One of our ministries while I was in school was pastoring a mountain church. Several people became Christians, and many others grew in the Lord. After seminary we moved to Newton, Kansas, where for six years the pattern of blessings continued. Then we pastored for nearly six years in the Wheaton, Illinois, area and twelve years in Urbana, Illinois.

In the twenty-five years Sally and I had been involved in pastoral and people-helping ministries prior to the discovery of Becki's cancer, we had watched God's supernatural restoration in thousands of people who had been healed from sin, made physically whole or rescued from serious financial or relational problems. We had participated as God rescued demon-possessed people or raised hundreds of thousands of dollars for missions.

We saw God turn humanly impossible situations into miraculous solutions, such as in the case of Mildred. She lived in one of our communities and was experiencing a very severe midlife transition. She was also apparently struggling with hormone imbalance. She was extremely depressed and suicidal. She had frequently attempted to take her life, and her husband was frantic. She had seen several doctors and had been hospitalized in three different hospitals. She also had received more than two dozen shock treatments and had undergone endless hours of psychiatric counseling. Nothing seemed to help. The doctors were at the end of their ropes.

Finally, one psychiatrist said to her, "We have tried everything, and yet we have not broken through this problem. I would suggest that you talk to your minister and receive his comfort."

## My Panic Prayer

Mildred was released from the hospital, and she knocked on my study door the next day. When she reported to me what the psychiatrist had said, I was so angry at him I wanted to strangle him. I was the ripe old age of twenty-seven, with very little training in counseling. How could he have the nerve to dump this woman in my lap!

I had been involved in her long, arduous struggle, but now it was left completely to me. She looked at me with pathetic eyes which pleaded an inaudible message, "Please help me."

As I listened to her story about her release from medical help, I silently poured out my heart to God, "Dear God, what am I to do? This woman's problem is far beyond my training and ability. I don't have the faintest clue of where to start or what to say. She is a hopeless victim. I, too, am just as helpless as she. Yet you have placed her in my care. Give me—give her—what we both need in these moments."

After she concluded her story and I had finished my cry for help to God, I was impressed by God that I should ask her how she would feel if she would die in the next few moments. I expected her to say that she would be relieved, that finally she could escape this torment. After all, she had attempted to take her life on many occasions.

Instead, terror was written across her face. It was as if her heart stopped beating and an anguished internal war raged within her. Yes, she wanted to die, but she was afraid of facing God after death.

In the minutes that followed, she poured out her fear of being judged by God and condemned to everlasting hell. She had been raised in the church and had given her life to Jesus Christ as her Lord and Savior. She had taught Sunday school and vacation Bible school classes and had served on numerous committees in various churches, but she was terrorized by the thought of death.

Her fear of being condemned to an endless hell not only shocked me, but caused me to inwardly question, "Why?" The words spilled out of my mind into audible speech, "Why are you afraid to die? I thought you were a Christian. Why are you afraid that God will send you to hell?"

## The Horrible Accident

In the next minutes she went back to a specific event in her life for which she felt a deep and oppressive guilt. Even though she had asked God a thousand times to forgive her, she had never felt forgiven. She was afraid that one incident would cause her to be sent to hell.

Not only was my curiosity aroused, but I also began to realize that this might be the "key" that would unlock the door and free her from the terror she had been experiencing these past years. She then recounted a horrible accident.

As a busy young mother, she had rushed out of her house one day to run an errand in the car. She knew that her children were playing in the area, but she thought she had looked carefully behind the car. As she hurriedly backed the car out of the driveway, she heard a horrible grinding sound along with the scream of a child.

In utter disbelief, she leaped from the car and looked underneath to discover the horrible reality that she had backed her car over her own child on a tricycle. The minutes seemed to stretch into hours before help arrived. The ambulance carried the dead body of her young child away, but she carried the grinding guilt from that day forward.

### Was Forgiveness Possible?

How could God forgive her? How could she ever forgive herself? In her mind, this was such a heinous sin that she deserved to spend eternity in hell. No matter how many things she did or how frequently she asked God to forgive her, she was inwardly convinced that God was going to condemn her to hell.

After her painful story had spilled out, I was prompted by God to treat her as a person who had never known anything about God's love and forgiveness. I said, "Let's assume for now that you are not a Christian and that you are not forgiven for this horrible thing. Let's start from that point."

In the next hours we explored what it meant to become a Christian, the nature of God, his relationship to us, how he longs to forgive us and the finality of his pardon. She then came to realize that when she asked God to forgive her, he really did forgive her. Any feelings of future guilt that she would experience would be false guilt generated from her memories.

Very simply, she confessed her sins to Christ, asked for his forgiveness and accepted his pardon as her present reality regardless of her future feelings.

We met frequently in the following weeks and months to reinforce the decision that she had made. It seemed as if she made a magical recovery. No, it wasn't magical—it was miraculous. This woman who had been totally non-functioning seemed to come back from the grave. She began to cook and care for the house. She took a part-time job and started to work in church again.

## It Won't Happen

Asking God for help and watching his miraculous interventions was such a normal pattern of our lives that after Dr. Kline left our home that evening, I stood with Becki in the kitchen and said, "Honey, I know this report sounds really bad, but I don't believe God is going to let you lose your leg. He's going to heal you." I smiled gently at her and gave her a hug. "It's going to be O.K., Honey." I didn't have the remotest reason to believe God would *not* heal the cancer in her leg.

As Becki has mentioned, our family was planning to take a spring vacation in Florida. The doctor wanted to do surgery right away, but he agreed to let her go if she had surgery as soon as we returned.

In the days before we left for Florida we telephoned and wrote to interested friends and relatives around the country, asking them to pray that God would intervene so that Becki would not lose her leg. We also wrote to missionary friends overseas, asking them to join in prayer.

Of course, our church groups were again urged to pray that Becki's leg might be healed. Many participated in a round-the-clock prayer vigil. Some people fasted and spent that time praying specifically for God to restore Becki's leg. The Board of Leadership and pastoral staff called for large group prayer times at the church two evenings a week.

We left for our Florida vacation a few days after the doctor's news about Becki's need for amputation. Our family, accompanied by Raewyn and Barbara's former roommate, used the motor home Raewyn's parents loaned us.

Our friends the Coxes were traveling with us in their motor home. We had driven straight through for twenty-two hours when we stopped at a rest area in northern Florida to have breakfast. It was a warm, balmy morning, and we were enjoying being away from the ice and cold in Illinois.

**Would She Ever Run Again?**
Sally and I prepared breakfast in the motor home while Becki and the other girls were out running around. A little creek about five feet wide ran past our area. I watched as Becki ran toward it, leaped in the air and easily cleared the stream, landing on the other side. Involuntarily, a question pushed into my conscious mind, "Would Becki ever do that again?"

That nagging question prompted me to go outside and run with her. I challenged Becki and the other girls to a short race over to the restroom building about forty yards away. I had run track in high school and college, and I was still pretty fast. I knew I didn't have endurance to beat them in anything longer, but maybe my quickness would make up the difference in this sprint. We took off. I gave it all I had, but as we neared the building, I glanced to my right and saw Becki digging with all her might as her strong legs powered her past me.

I gave her a hug and that nagging question came back, "Would she ever run again?" I pushed the question out of my mind. Of course, she'd run again! God had answered hundreds of prayers. Certainly he was going to demonstrate his power, as he had so often in the past, and heal Becki's leg.

We arrived at a terrific location on Fort Myers Beach on the western side of Florida. We parked in a small grove of pine trees about a hundred feet from the ocean. The water was beautiful. We had fun sailing our sixteen-foot catamaran that we had towed from Illinois. It was relaxing to walk along the beach, trying to select the very best shells from the millions spread out before us. We tried to pack in as much life as possible in those few days.

Every time I looked at Becki, I wondered when God was going to act. Would it be now while we were here on vacation, or would it be when she was actually admitted to the hospital? Or would God wait to perform the miracle on the operating table, just moments before her leg was to be removed?

Each morning before starting the day, we spent time reading Scripture and praying for God to heal Becki's leg. The prayer was repeated at each meal and in personal quiet times with God. Again, as we dropped off to sleep we would pray, "God, please, heal Becki. Restore her leg. Demonstrate your power to people who don't believe that prayer works." Each day we were closer to "the showdown." Many times I said, "Hey, God, you can perform your miracle anytime now."

## Down to the Wire

After we returned home and Becki had completed her pre-surgical tests, we gathered around her hospital bed and again, as a family, prayed that Becki's leg would be healed. When we finished praying, I asked Becki if the lump was still there. She slid her hand down to the area just above her knee, felt for a moment, and then looked up at me and nodded, "It's still there."

"Well," I thought to myself, "this is no big problem because

God has bailed us out at the last minute thousands of times before. This is going to be one of those dramatic times when it goes right down to the wire. She will be wheeled off to the operating room, placed on the table, with the surgeon ready to perform the surgery. Then suddenly he will discover she has been healed. The surgical process will be stopped. Everyone will be amazed! We will praise God and live happily ever after." It all seemed so clear in my mind.

We were at the hospital early the next morning. I talked to Scott, the surgeon, and asked him to check carefully for the tumor before he started the surgical process. I expected God to come through with his last-minute miracle. Scott promised he would look closely.

In her hospital room Becki was lying flat on her back with a sheet covering her body. She was fully alert since she had requested not to have any pre-surgical medication. I looked at her pretty face, her twinkling eyes and her brave smile. I also looked at the sheet draped over her two strong legs. What would the sheet look like when I saw her next?

# Part II

# LIFE
# TAKES

# 5

## A FATHER'S PERSPECTIVE

# DARK DAY OF DESPAIR

**I** *remember the scene so clearly. I also easily relive* the strange combination of emotions—fear, hope, anticipation and deep despair.

Becki was wheeled out of her hospital room through the rear hallway and into the surgical elevator. The nurse pushed the button for the surgical floor and the doors closed.

Our family was separated. Becki was on her way to surgery, either to discover that God had healed her or to have her leg amputated. Sally, Barbara, Brenda and I found our way to the waiting room, which was packed with friends who had come to pray and encourage us during this crisis. So many people had come that they spilled over into two other waiting rooms.

It was a strange situation for me. I tried to wear several "hats" at the same moment. I was pastor, husband, father and myself. Some people had come to encourage us, so I wore the hat of a recipient. Other people needed to hear a word of encouragement from me, so for them I put on my pastoral hat. At the same time, I was trying to wear the hat of caregiver for my family. Somewhere in the middle were my own needs. What was going to happen? When would God pull off his miracle?

## The Confrontation

Such a large crowd of friends had gathered at the hospital that the waiting-room attendant indignantly confronted me. "Why did you allow all of these people to come here?" she asked. "These waiting rooms are so crowded that it is difficult for me to do my job. You must send some of the people away now!"

I exploded, "My daughter's up there in surgery. She may be having her leg amputated at this very moment! Yet all you can worry about is whether your working conditions are right!" I was *very* angry.

Sally tried to calm me. "Jim," she whispered, "she doesn't understand; don't let her bother you." Some of the leaders of the church moved in to smooth the situation. But the attendant seemed unmoved and demanded again that the people leave.

Her demand further enraged me. I told her sarcastically, "You're right. Hospitals and people like you are only here to be served by patients and their families. You're not here to serve us."

With that I walked out into a hallway. Some of the church leaders again stepped in and quieted the woman by assuring her that part of the group would move to other areas of the hospital.

I had moved to the stark white hall, trying to gain my composure. What was happening up in surgery? I glanced at my watch. Forty-five minutes . . . then an hour . . . still no word from surgery. It doesn't take this long to examine the leg and verify the miracle.

For the first time, I began to face the reality that Becki was probably having her leg amputated. No miracle of healing had taken place. My heart began to sink.

The next hours were a blur. We moved from area to area in the hospital, comforting and being comforted by the people who had come to be with us. As the minutes ticked by, I felt the growing reality that Becki had actually lost her leg. I tried to put all the questions out of my mind. Maybe this was all a bad dream. Maybe I would wake up to find Becki running on both legs.

### I'm Sorry. . .

Two hours and forty-five minutes had passed when suddenly Scott, our doctor, appeared in the barren corridor where Sally and I were walking with our other two daughters. He pulled off his green hat as he walked directly toward me. He looked squarely into my face and said, "I'm sorry—we had to take Becki's leg."

I was stunned. My mind was a jumble of confusion, questions and shocked disbelief. Scott explained that her left leg had been amputated more than halfway up her thigh. He was talking—but I was in a numbed trance.

"I'm positive that we got all of the cancer because the bone samples from the upper end of the surgical area tested out as normal bone," he continued. "She is in the recovery room now and is doing very well. She is a very strong young woman."

Then he repeated, "I'm sorry it had to happen—but it looks like we got all of the cancer."

Scott and Sally talked a bit more, but I was in a daze. I was angry. Where was God? Why did he answer so many other prayers, which by comparison seemed inconsequential, but now he had turned a deaf ear?

Scott turned and walked away. The four of us were alone again at the end of that cold, sterile hallway. In my anguish, I started beating on the wall and crying out loudly, "Where is God? Doesn't he care?" Then I wheeled around and said to Sally, "Well, we are really on our own. From now on, we will just have to take care of ourselves. God doesn't seem to be taking care of us anymore."

## The Grisly Retreat

I turned and stumbled away from Sally and the two girls. I needed to be totally alone. I walked the familiar corridors of the hospital, looking for a place to hide with my awful heartache. I came to one of the elevators which I had frequently used on previous pastoral errands of mercy.

This time I pushed the button for the basement. The elevator took me to the bowels of the hospital. The door opened on an empty corridor. This was the ideal place to be alone. The hall was dimly lighted. No one was around. I wouldn't have to face all of those people upstairs. What could I say to them anyway? Many of them were new Christians. Should I just smile and say, "Prayer doesn't work. God let us down"?

I turned a corner onto another hallway and sat down on a bench. This place was *very* familiar in a grisly sort of way. It was the morgue.

I had been here some months before to identify the body of a young woman who had killed herself because her husband was having an affair. She had died from a drug overdose. Three days had passed before they found her bloated body in her car in an isolated cornfield. She had a note pinned on her blouse for her husband. It said, "You win."

I remembered her face as the coroner pulled back the sheet. It had a frightening, black appearance. I became sick to my stomach as I looked at her and realized that she had given up hope. She was one of my counselees, a Christian from a Christian home. But no miracle had happened for her, and she took her life.

## The Anguish

In those hours, as I sat outside the morgue after Becki's amputation, I could understand why that woman in her state of hopelessness had committed suicide. I, too, wished that I could quickly slip into eternity.

I understood how Job felt as he said,

"Let the day of my birth be cursed. . . . Let that day be forever forgotten. Let it be lost to God, shrouded in eternal darkness" (Job 3:3-4, LB).

Job continued pouring out his heart in anguish,

"Why didn't I die at birth? Why did the midwife let me live? . . . Oh, to have been stillborn! to have never breathed or seen the light . . . . Why is a man allowed to be born if God is only going to give him a hopeless life of uselessness and frustration? . . . What I've always feared has happened to me. I was not fat and lazy, yet trouble struck me down" (vv. 11-12, 16, 25-26, LB).

Job was not spiritually fat or lazy. In fact, God's description of him was that "he is the finest man in all the earth—a good man who fears God and will have nothing to do with evil" (Job 1:8, LB). Yet Job was swept under with a test that seemed too great to bear. He wanted to die.

I had read the book of Job many times and had preached

sermons from it. But now his experiences were different to me—I was *with* Job in his anguish.

I felt emotionally and spiritually as if I had been run over by a cement truck. I was angry, crushed with disappointment, confused, in despair and lonely for my best friend—God. But he seemed to have abandoned me.

## The Reality

Sally had urged me to be waiting for Becki when she was brought back from the recovery room. So I returned upstairs. As I walked into Becki's room, she wasn't back yet. Though the room was full of flowers, plants, cards and assorted stuffed animals, it felt empty and cold. I stood near the bed and waited for Becki to be wheeled in.

What would I say to her? Could I ever apologize for God? How could I tell her I was sorry for leading her astray about God healing her? My sense of betrayal was tearing me apart.

I was totally unprepared for what was to happen next. We stood back as Becki was wheeled into the room. The nurses went about their duties of checking the IV and various other tubes attached to her.

I was at the head of the bed on Becki's left side. After the nurse on my side of the bed finished her tasks, she turned to me and said, "O.K." Then she stepped back. For the first time my eyes saw what my heart had dreaded.

Becki's golden hair was spread out over the pillow. The clean white sheet was pulled up under her armpits. I saw the IV tube connected to her left arm. My eye quickly went to the right side of her body. I followed the contour of her body all the way down her right leg. The sheet was raised, clearly showing the outline of her right leg with her toes pointing to the ceiling.

My eyes came back to her waist. I felt sick to my stomach as I followed the contour of the sheet down her left leg. About six inches below her groin the sheet fell flat to the bed. There was nothing—nothing where her left leg should have been.

Then, mercifully, a great, cold numbness settled over me. In my new non-feeling state, I quit worrying about my theological questions, my promises to Becki or even whether God existed. What was most important at this moment was to help Becki. I wanted to let her know how deeply I loved her—how we all loved her.

Becki stirred, smiled, took hold of our hands and said, "Hi." There wasn't one trace of anger, bitterness or confusion in her. Her face expressed a deep, settled peace, indicating that she knew God was in all of this.

## The Encouragement

During those days of recovery in the hospital, I watched Becki with amazement. Repeatedly, she put people at ease. Classmates who came to visit would avoid looking at her stump, discussing everything except her amputation. Becki, however, immediately helped people feel comfortable. She joked about how she had lost seventeen pounds in three hours. Or she encouraged them to look at her basketball-size stump.

Becki's positive attitude was healing for me. I never had to apologize for God or tell her that I was sorry for promising her that she would not lose her leg.

She had so completely dealt with the amputation before it happened that her life was as steady as a grandfather clock. The amputation never caused her to miss a beat.

Her stability and confidence in God was probably the major force that brought me through the whole ordeal. "After all," I thought to myself, "she was the one who lost her leg. If she could trust God, maybe sometime I could also trust him again."

During those next days, my emotions felt like the ocean waves. Sometimes, as when a wave has just gone out, everything seemed calm. But other times, as when the incoming wave crashes at the crest, my emotions were almost uncontrollable. At those times I had to get out of Becki's hospital room to regain my composure.

## The Anger

I was upset by the easy answers of people trying to console me. An incident happened two days after Becki's surgery that showed how wounded and vulnerable I was. Sally and I were spending most of our time with Becki in the hospital, but that day we left briefly to go to a nearby restaurant for a quick lunch. As we were being led to our seats, we passed a table of concerned friends. The man on the end reached out and grabbed hold of my sleeve.

I turned, expecting only to give him a casual greeting. Instead he shocked me by announcing, "Jim, I know *why* God allowed Becki's leg to be amputated." I didn't want to hear what he was going to say, but he hung on to my coat sleeve.

Then his awful answer spilled out, "God has used Becki's amputation to bring about a revival in our church and in other Christians. People have really learned to pray and have become serious in their walk with God. This has caused a spiritual awakening in our city."

I'm sure he didn't realize how his words were affecting me, but the anger within me was white-hot. I was ready to explode. I asked him a question, with as much control as I could muster, "How long does a revival last?" Without waiting for him to answer, I spewed out my sarcastic answer, "Most church revivals only last three to six months. Then what does God do? Chop off Becki's other leg so that the church can be revived again? Then does he take one arm and finally her other arm? There isn't enough of Becki to keep any church alive spiritually."

With that, I spun around and went on to our table far in the back of the restaurant. I kept telling myself that he really wanted to help. But the reality was that his attempt at providing answers had only made my problem greater.

I was in deep trouble. I was very angry, crushed that God had not answered my prayer and the prayers of thousands of other people. I lashed out at almost anybody who came near to me, reacting many times as if I were a snarling, wounded, wild animal.

Becki had dozens and dozens of visitors. Certain visitors, however, sent my emotions tumbling. Cheerleaders or girls from the track team really bothered me. I looked at their healthy bodies and realized that Becki would never again do what these girls could do with ease. It seemed so unfair. Becki not only had been a good athlete but she was a terrific spiritual leader. Why was she cut down?

I had to get out of her room. It was better for me to walk the hospital halls, glancing into the rooms of sick people, than to think about the healthy bodies of Becki's friends.

I also needed to get out of the room when Becki was visited by "Pollyanna" Christians. These people came in with their painted-on Christian smiles. They had a Bible verse for every problem. They would slap me on the back and say, "Cheer up, brother." (They always use the word *brother*.) "All things work together for good," they'd say.

I not only got out of the room when these people came, but I also had to fight the urge to vomit. Why didn't God keep these people away? It was as if these "Job's helpers" came to rub my face in my failure.

## What Now?

Each time I had to leave the room or each time the giant wave of emotional despair swept over me, I wondered about my future. Would I ever again preach? How could I? I wished that I were a plumber. I could continue to fix pipes whether God was alive or dead, whether prayer was answered or not. But I was the senior pastor of a *Bible* church. Week by week I taught the Bible. I had repeatedly told people, "God loves you and has a wonderful plan for your life." But now I sarcastically exclaimed to myself, *"So this is God's wonderful plan!"*

I began to think of alternative ways to make a living. I wondered what I could do that would enable me to get away from every Christian and anything that reminded me of God. I concluded that God was either impotent, didn't care, or he was dead. These were truly the darkest days of my life. Becki had lost her leg. I had lost God. Now I wished for death.

# 6

## A MOTHER'S PERSPECTIVE

# A DIFFERENT KIND OF MIRACLE

**W**hile I absent-mindedly chatted with our friends in the waiting room, I was silently talking with the Lord about what might be happening to Becki in the operating room. Suddenly I became aware that Jim and the woman in charge of the waiting room were having an argument. She was saying we had too many visitors and demanded that most of them leave so that we met the requirement of four people per patient.

I was embarrassed that Jim was losing his temper with this woman, but I was also aggravated at her for being so insensitive to us. Yes, we had more visitors in the room than anyone else, but only two or three other patients had someone waiting for them that morning. Those people didn't seem to mind that we had a big group. Our friends had been talking quietly among themselves or sitting silently. After all the couches and chairs had been taken, our visitors sat on the floor. We weren't causing a problem to anyone except the lady who had a quota to maintain.

Now where should we go? No other place in the hospital had enough room for our group. If we split up, Jim and I couldn't be in every place with them. Where would the doctor find us after surgery? We had told him we would be in this waiting room.

I don't know where our friends went. I just remember that Jim, Barbara, Brenda and I were separated from everyone else, ending up in an empty room with no furniture. It looked as if it were being remodeled. We sat down on some clumps of partially rolled carpet and alternately prayed aloud, talked and stared at the walls that needed to be repainted.

Even though this was an ugly place at an ugly moment, I was glad that we could be together. Brenda was home from Taylor University, and Barbara, who was attending the University of Illinois, was also missing her classes to be with us. We were joined together in our earnest desire for God to surround Becki with his love, whatever he was allowing to happen.

I remember Brenda saying, "I know we've had a lot of hard times in our family lately, but aren't we glad they are just physical problems? Here we are—we all love each other and we're all Christians who are walking with the Lord. One of us isn't off rebelling somewhere. We may have all sorts of physical problems (as she looked at Barbara encased in an upper body cast due to her broken collar bone), but we are united as a family under the Lord."

## On Our Own?

When we thought it was time to hear from Dr. Kline that he had discovered the amputation wasn't necessary, we moved out into a hallway where he could find us. He didn't come. We stood around in the empty, impersonal hall for what seemed like endless hours.

When Dr. Kline finally did come, he told us with great anguish that he had amputated Becki's leg. We listened numbly to his explanation. I had hoped he would tell us Becki still had her leg because the tumor had disappeared, but I wasn't surprised when his news was the opposite. I was relieved that Becki had made it through the surgery very well and that he was confident all the malignant area was removed. I was also glad that the tumor had still been confined within the bone wall so that the cancer most likely had not spread.

One of us quickly related the news to our waiting friends, and then the four of us retreated into a more isolated hall to wait until we could see Becki in her room. That section of the hospital was to undergo reconstruction soon. There seemed to be no light, or perhaps the darkness I remember was in my soul. I recall sitting on a bench while Jim paced the floor.

Suddenly Jim stopped pacing and faced me. With his jaw set, he looked into my eyes and said, "We need to be very strong now. We'll have to get through this time on our own. It's obvious that God isn't going to help us." I reached out to touch him, but he walked off and around a corner.

I didn't agree that God had abandoned us. I was very sorry Jim was so profoundly disappointed that God hadn't healed Becki, but I believed God knew what he was doing. God had always taken care of us and he still would.

I desperately wanted to comfort Jim, but he had walked out of sight. I felt pulled in two directions, but I decided not to follow him since I wanted to be where the nurse could find us to tell us we could see Becki. I was agonizing about the tremendous pain I thought she would be suffering. Were the nurses and attendants in the recovery room doing everything they could to make her comfortable? I was anxious to be with her.

As I sat there waiting, I wondered what the medical staff was doing right then with that precious leg they had removed. Had they put it in a plastic bag for the trash collection? Were they cramming it into an incinerator? Were they cutting it up for scientific study? Was someone admiring how shapely and tanned it was? Those thoughts hurt too much! I abruptly shoved them out of my mind and went back into "neutral" until we could see Becki again.

## The Shock

No one came for us, so eventually we went to see if Becki had been returned to her room yet. She wasn't back when we walked in, but her bed with clean, tightly tucked sheets was ready for her. Cards and gifts that had arrived were sitting around the room.

I could tell that Jim was depressed and quietly angry. He kept saying, "I can't take this. I have to get out of here." I found it hard to understand why he would want to leave when Becki needed us so much.

Soon a nurse came and asked us to leave the room so that the gurney carrying Becki could be rolled next to her bed. She drew the drape that separated Becki's bed from her roommate's section. As I stepped into the hall, I saw the gurney. I was totally unprepared for what I saw.

Becki was whiter than her sheets. I had seen her after four other surgeries and numerous accidents, but never had she looked so pale. I was stunned. For the first time, I thought of her in connection with death.

And that terrible flat spot on the gurney! Her left leg was *definitely gone.*

For a split second, I wanted to bolt. I was standing by a door that led to a back stairway. I felt as if I were being pulled to the door by an unseen force. I could envision myself just disappearing.

That feeling left as quickly as it came. I wouldn't run; everyone needed me now. I was shocked that I would even have had such a thought, but I did. And now I better understood some of Jim's struggles.

## Mother on Guard

I followed the gurney into Becki's room and stood by helplessly while the attendants moved her onto her bed. One of them let go of her before the other one did, and her body jolted as she dropped. They then had to shift her to get her centered in the bed. With each move, Becki groaned a little.

Like a mother bear, I wanted to growl at them. I was angry that they weren't more gentle. I felt like snarling, "This girl has just had her leg removed. Be careful with her!"

Nurses were standing around getting all her tubes adjusted. After they checked her vital signs, they left for a moment and we were alone with Becki. She reached out one hand and with a weak, but perky, little grin said, "Hi."

She was still Becki! They hadn't amputated her spirit. She still had her wit and courage.

We patted her and told her we loved her. We let her know that Dr. Kline felt sure he had removed all of the cancer. We couldn't keep our eyes off the huge ball where her left leg had been amputated. She helped us check it out as we carefully lifted the sheet. All we saw was a tremendous mass of wrappings! The stump was already greatly swollen and, with miles of bandages around it, it looked bigger than a basketball. No one had prepared us for shocking little details like this.

As soon as a lull occurred in the conversation or activity around her bed, Becki would fall asleep. A few selected visitors tip-toed in to see her that afternoon. She roused when they entered and tried to talk to them, but soon she'd start mumbling and slurring her words as she drowsed off again.

Jim, Barbara, Brenda and I took turns standing beside Becki. We stroked her forehead, patted her arms and tried to show that we cared for her very much. We wanted somehow to ease her pain. Nurses continued to come and go, keeping a close watch on her blood pressure, pulse and other vital functions.

I stayed in her room constantly. I was aware that friends were still at the hospital, sending their greetings into the room with nurses or family members. More flowers kept arriving. We also got word that friends from around the nation were telephoning our home for news of whether or not she had to have the amputation.

## Midnight Watch

Late that evening the rest of the family went home, and I prepared for the night shift with Becki. The nurses hauled in a strange, old plastic lounge chair for me to rest on when I didn't need to be at Becki's bedside.

I was dozing on that old couch when I heard Becki stir. "Mom, what time is it?" she asked. My watch showed that it was close to midnight.

I got up to stand beside her. I couldn't imagine how intense the pain must be. I wished that I could experience her pain for her. Why couldn't I have lost my leg instead of her?

"Mom, please tell them not to give me any more morphine. I think I can stand the pain with just some pain pills," she said clearly.

I couldn't believe it! Dr. Kline had warned us that she might need to be heavily sedated for three or four days; then we probably could ease off to lighter medication.

"Are you sure?" I asked.

"I'm sure," she declared. "I really feel that God is right here in a special way, helping me take this pain."

## Amazingly Remodeled

We were continually surprised by Becki's speedy recovery. God enabled her to be ahead of schedule on every milestone her medical team had for her. She not only required less pain medication than expected, but she was also able to be up and around the hospital very quickly.

The day after surgery the physical therapist came to her room. The first day's task was to sit up and move out of bed into a wheelchair. Becki did that easily without any help. So the therapist said, "Well, we can just go right on to Lesson Two, which is to take you to the therapy room." So she wheeled Becki down to Physical Therapy.

The therapist rolled Becki into the room and left her sitting in the wheelchair while she walked out to get something. Becki noticed a large mirror on the opposite wall. Since she hadn't yet seen herself full-length, she thought, "Now is my chance to see how other people will see me." She stood up to get a better view.

She was dressed in one of those stunning hospital gowns and a Tedd hose (a white elasticized stocking to keep the blood circulating in her good leg while in bed). Her stump was wrapped with an ace bandage. It was very swollen and, with the bandage, was tremendously out of proportion to the rest of her body.

She was standing with her arms crossed, studying how much of her leg had been taken off, when the physical therapist walked back in. Becki asked, "Well, what are we supposed to be doing down here? Am I supposed to lift weights or some-thing?"

Without looking up from the papers she held, the therapist said, "I want you to learn to balance on one foot using the parallel bars for support." Then she turned to give Becki eye contact. "Oh!" she stammered, "you're already standing and perfectly balanced without the bars!"

The next day when the physical therapist came, she said, "Well, since you've already demonstrated good balance, we'll teach you to walk with crutches." What she didn't know was that Becki had already used her crutches from home to make a trip around the hospital floor. She had just climbed back into bed before the therapist came in. Unwittingly, Becki had com-pleted Lesson Three. That's when the therapist discharged her from therapy until she would start gait training as an outpa-tient with an artificial leg.

## What's Wrong with Her?
Becki was a congenial hostess to all who came to see her. Three days after surgery an entire high-school chemistry class came to visit. The hospital gave them a conference room to use. She entertained the class from her wheelchair. Her cheery attitude was a boost to all the rest of us.

Becki's positive reaction didn't always produce positive re-sponses in others, however, especially one nurse. The hospital used a "primary health care" system, which was to have one registered nurse give the total care for a patient, instead of many nurses and aids each giving portions of the care. Becki's primary nurse was sure that Becki's enthusiastic manner meant that she wasn't facing her situation honestly.

"If she'd just cry or be angry, I'd know she was handling this more realistically," the nurse said to me as she drew me aside into a separate room. "It is absolutely unnatural not to be depressed about such a loss. She needs to grieve! Are you sure she isn't pretending to be strong in order to help you and your husband cope?"

I tried to assure the nurse that I felt Becki was very aware of what had happened to her and what the outlook was for her future. Our family had talked thoroughly about all that this surgery and possible chemotherapy would entail. I explained to the nurse, "God seems to have given her an unusual ability to deal with her circumstances." This concept further confirmed the nurse's suspicions that this was a strange family!

That nurse did not come back to work during the rest of Becki's hospitalization. Another nurse told us, "She just couldn't handle having Becki as a patient. Seeing someone so young go through a tragic amputation was too much for her. And then to have Becki to be so 'up' about it was the last straw. She's taking some vacation days."

## Surprise, Doctor!

I had never seen so many huge stuffed bears and dogs except in store displays. Now they were in Becki's hospital room. Two of the stuffed animals were five feet high. Flowers filled every window ledge and table top. I think the doctor released her early because he no longer could locate her in the room. When it was time to take Becki home, Jim and I each drove a car filled with gifts. She and her crutches were buried somewhere in one of the cars.

We had prepared the living room couch as her convalescent bed. That way she could be in the center of the family's activities, and visitors could easily come and go. I thought she might be on the couch for weeks, but God continued to help her make a remarkable rebound to her former lifestyle.

Becki was eager to get back to school, but Dr. Kline wanted her to go slowly since she was recovering from major surgery.

The school made arrangements for a "homebound instructor" to come to our house so that she could keep up with her classes. In a few days Becki was frustrated because the instructor wasn't knowledgeable about every subject. Becki felt the tutoring just wasted time. Besides, she was missing her friends and the hustle–bustle of high–school life.

When Dr. Kline learned that Becki had already been in several public places—shopping malls, a volleyball tournament, a high–school track event and church—he decided that returning to school would not be a big problem. Fewer than three weeks after surgery she started easing back into the school schedule by attending two or three hours at a time.

I stood by Becki the first Sunday she went to church, which was twelve days after surgery. As we rose to sing a hymn, I marveled at her perfect balance. Through the entire song, she stood perfectly still on one leg. I was the one teetering around!

Becki's stump was bandaged for several weeks, but the swelling was gradually going down. We had to keep fresh dressings on the incision. One day as we put on a clean bandage before Becki's first follow–up visit with Dr. Kline, we couldn't resist creating a surprise for him. When she unwrapped the bandage for him in his office, he shook his head. Above the big smile–shaped incision on the end of her stump were a marking–pen nose and eyes to complete the smiley face!

### The Rest of Her Life

Dr. Kline had good news for us at one of our visits. He and the other specialists from around the nation had decided that Becki would not need chemotherapy. Becki was very relieved; she had been dreading the prospects of nausea, hair loss and other side effects from such treatment. We were all glad for the good indication that the cancer was gone.

Dr. Kline warned us, however, that because of the rare type of malignancy, Becki would need to be tested periodically for the next fifteen years instead of the usual five. (With each passing year that she has received "a clean bill of health," we have felt deep gratitude to the Lord for the life and health he is giving Becki.)

In the early months after her amputation, I would look at Becki's stump and say to myself, "Just think, she's going to be like this for the rest of her life." As soon as I would say the word *life,* I would reprimand myself and add, *"But she does have her life!"*

Shortly after her amputation, she was put in touch with two other teen-agers who recently had had a leg removed because of cancer. Each of those kids, however, also had malignant tumors in other parts of their bodies. The prognosis for them was grim.

In both cases Jim and I visited the parents. We encouraged them about all their teen could do as an amputee, but we could not encourage them that their child had a long life to live. We grieved for them and were humbled to think that God had chosen to spare Becki's life. In addition, he had made it a vivacious, abundant one.

It was true that Becki no longer had her left leg. But one day in those early weeks of adjustment to life on one leg, Becki said, "God promises to give me everything I need. If I needed two legs, he wouldn't have taken one away."

No, God had not performed a physical healing before the amputation. But it soon was evident that he had given her exceptional physical recovery after the surgery and had performed remarkable spiritual and emotional miracles in her.

# 7

# IT REALLY
# HAPPENED

**T**he next thing I remember was waking up in terrible pain. I was so groggy that I couldn't sit up to see if my left leg was there. I tried to move it. All I felt was incredible pain. "O.K., God, it really has happened," I thought. "Here we go."

In that very first minute, as the nurse offered me something more for the pain, I knew I was representing God. Christ was in me, and I wanted his power to show through me even in that difficult moment. I didn't want the pain to get the best of me and make me a crabby patient. I had always been Christ's representative, but I realized people were going to notice me more now because I had only one leg. I sensed the call to be his ambassador.

## New Day—New Life

After I was out of the recovery room and back in my room, a barrage of school kids, church friends and other visitors came to support me and my parents. Later I was told that so many visitors came, the nurses became frustrated trying to screen them. They put a sign on my door, asking people to limit their visits. Even then the hall was crowded with friends waiting to get in.

The first day after surgery is just a hazy memory. I was groggy from the anesthesia and morphine and kept falling asleep. I would waken briefly and feel embarrassed that I wasn't talking to all these people who had come. I kept apologizing, "I'm sorry I'm not being very polite. . . ." Then I'd fall asleep right in the middle of my sentence.

The first time I was fully conscious came in the middle of the night. The anesthesia had worn off and I was reasonably alert. I woke up to a dim light in the room. The night nurse was checking my vital signs.

Now that the fuzziness from the anesthesia was gone, the reality that I actually had lost my leg was very vivid. I asked myself, "Where do I go from here? How do I start this next day? After all, I've never been disabled before." I wondered how people would treat me and if I really would be able to deal with being an amputee. This new day would *definitely* be different from any I had ever had in my life. My mom was in the room, lying on a makeshift couch next to my bed. When she noticed I was awake, she got up and stood next to me. She talked with me and reaffirmed that God would use this amputation. "God had a reason for allowing this to happen," she said. "He has a special plan and is preparing you to do something remarkable." Her assurance helped keep me focused and to anticipate God's work during the next few hours and days.

I increasingly realized that God *had* chosen me to do something special. I certainly didn't know *what* he had planned, but I knew he would use me. I had always known God had a design for my life, as he does for us all. Now he was showing me what that design looked like—it was one-legged. I felt honored and excited that he had given me the privilege to serve him in a very unique way.

## A Remodeled Body

God gave me a remarkably fast recovery, and I knew it was a special gift from him. I progressed quickly in the physical therapy program so that in a couple of days I was walking on crutches, feeling relatively stable.

My hospital floor was circular, with a nurses' station in the middle. As I walked around, I looked in the rooms at other patients, most of whom were cancer victims. I saw older people who were suffering with great pain. I met a twelve-year-old girl who didn't have long to live. She and her family were devastated.

As I compared my circumstances with those of other patients, I knew I was greatly blessed. My doctors were quite positive that my surgery had cured me. They still hadn't decided whether I should have chemotherapy, but they were very confident that the amputation was a large part of the treatment.

## Different But Not Different

The first few days after surgery were not only a time for physical recovery but also for my social adjustment. When my friends came into my hospital room, I could sense their discomfort. They wanted to encourage me and show they were thinking about me, but my missing leg distressed them. It wasn't just knee surgery that would heal in a few weeks. They knew that I was now permanently changed physically.

Many of my friends were afraid my amputation would alter my personality. They were unsure how I would react, so when they came to see me, they would awkwardly look out the window, at my parents or at the cards and flowers—anywhere but the vacant spot on my bed. They stood around, shuffling their feet, not knowing what to do or say. So I joked with them or invited them to sit down on the empty side of the bed. Sitting on the bed where my left leg should have been, helped them accept the obvious and realize I was the same person as before.

They seemed surprised to find me cheerful, interested in what they were doing and involved in life. Often I made wisecracks about what a great diet I was on: "Look, I lost seventeen pounds in three hours." Or I'd joke about the hospital expenses: "You know, it cost an arm and a leg to be in here, but the insurance covered the arm." I wanted to let them know they didn't need to be afraid or embarrassed.

## Helping the Able-bodied

I realized early that if I got people over the initial barrier of my missing leg, our interaction would be more normal. I tried to handle their questions and uncomfortableness right away so that they could stop being worried about my one-leggedness or my obvious prosthesis. If they became too caught up in the fact that I was different, I would use puns to ease the situation, such as "I can't stand on my own two feet." Or "I eat like I have a hollow leg."

I needed to be an educator to the able-bodied people around me. I had been "normal" for sixteen years, and I knew how I had perceived disabled people. I could remember being un-comfortable around people in wheelchairs, on crutches or with an unusual gait. I had wanted to ask questions but was em-barrassed. Suddenly, after a three-hour surgery, I was "dis-abled." Now that I was on the other side of the fence, I could help able-bodied people understand that disabled people are very normal, with similar struggles as theirs.

As a child, I was very curious about the disabled. When we lived in Carol Stream, Illinois, a man in our church had lost his arm as a child in a farm accident. He didn't wear a prosthetic limb, so he always had an empty sleeve. When he wore a suit coat, he would tuck the sleeve into his pocket. When I was three or four years old, I desperately wanted to peek up his empty sleeve and see what it looked like not to have an arm. Were little fingers up there or what? Of course, I didn't ask the man, or any other disabled person, my questions.

Now within hours I had become one of those "handicapped" people. I knew people were curious but didn't know what to say, so I deliberately started conversations about my amputation. I answered tons of questions. Similar to being the Shell Answer Man, I was the "Gimp Answer Woman"—all you ever wanted to know about the disabled but were afraid to ask. It was an advantage for me to understand what people might be feeling. I realized that many thought I would become weird, withdrawn and self-conscious. They expected me to be embarrassed about my stump or ashamed to be seen on crutches. Some people thought I should stay at home until I got an artificial leg and looked "presentable." I would have a limp because of my pros-thesis, but that would be more appropriate—according to them—than going around with one leg and a stump.

**Learning Everything Again**
Five days after my amputation, I was discharged from the hos-

pital. Going home meant learning to do many things differently. Much of what I had taken sixteen years to learn now had to be relearned. The first time around I had learned gradually and according to my age and ability. Now, suddenly, everything had to be done a new way all at once: walking, dressing, getting in and out of the bathtub, carrying a glass of water or my school books, walking up steps on crutches without falling backwards.

My two limiting factors were pain and endurance. I still had my stitches and my stump was quite swollen. The stump was very painful if I bounced too much or put pressure on it. My endurance was low because of the trauma of surgery and the resulting inactivity. I perspired heavily with the slightest exertion. Getting to the bathroom and back was a major feat.

Mom and Dad urged me to call for help when I needed something. But I was sixteen and didn't want to be dependent upon them. I was feeling almost like an adult; I wanted to do everything I could for myself. So I carried things my own way by scooting along on the floor from room to room. Hopping still hurt my incision too much.

**Hey, Mom!**
I could hardly wait to get going again. I tried to rest and re-cuperate the first week after my amputation, but one day when Mom wasn't paying attention, I went outside into our backyard. I got up in the old tree fort that Dad and I had built when I was younger. After climbing into the fort, I continued up into the tree branches for about thirty feet. I was thrilled as I realized that my three limbs could still do plenty. I was able to maneuver up a ladder and even up a tree!

I was so excited, I yelled, "Mom, Mom, come out and see me!" She rushed out and about had a heart attack when she saw where I was. She must have thought I was going to fall and ruin the healthy body parts I still had. I was only trying to find out what my body could do.

## My "Comforter"

One night a student from the University of Illinois came to talk to me. He had a below-the-knee amputation and walked with a noticeable limp. I'm not sure how he learned about me, but apparently his reason for coming was to talk to me about life as an amputee and what to expect from an artificial leg.

Soon I realized everything he said was negative. He complained about the pain from his artificial leg and his dreadful phantom pain (feeling as if the amputated limb is still there, which *can be* excruciating). Girls didn't like him, he couldn't do this and he couldn't do that. Eventually I asked, "Well, what about the bright side? Has there been anything good?" He was so dismal and felt so persecuted because of his handicap that I ended up trying to encourage *him*.

I felt sorry that he had problems living with his amputation, but I vowed I would *never* be like that! I determined not to grump about my situation nor complain about the things I couldn't do. I was going to look for all the things I *could* do.

## "I Can Do It!"

That impetus carried me into the next several weeks and helped me try many activities. It was a challenge to see how many things I could do, instead of automatically ruling them out. I tried everything from driving a car (which wasn't hard with an automatic transmission and my remaining right leg) to lugging my backpack full of books up and down stairs at school or pushing a supermarket shopping cart while on crutches and one leg.

I hadn't yet been fitted with an artificial leg. That was to come in about three-and-a-half months after my stump had shrunk. Rather than give me a temporary pylon (peg leg) first, they decided to fit me with a permanent prosthesis as soon as my stump was in a suitable condition. In the meantime, I wanted to live as normally as possible.

During my first week back at school, I went to my physical education class. My teacher just assumed I wouldn't want to participate, since many girls looked for every opportunity to get out of a class that messed up their hair and make-up. However, I couldn't wait to see what I could do. My classmates were amazed that I could play volleyball without my prosthesis or crutches. I hopped around, sometimes hitting the ball and sometimes missing, just like anyone else. After a couple of minutes, my classmates quit gawking and realized I was still like any other girl in most ways.

When I went to the prom about six weeks after my surgery, I surprised the people who thought I'd drop out and become a recluse. I still didn't have my artificial leg, but I danced by standing in one place, with my date pivoting around me. We both had a great time!

## The Reason for the Difference

My amputation showed me the unbalanced emphasis our society puts on our physical bodies. Many of my friends thought that if they were in my shoes—or shoe, I should say—they would have withdrawn. Girlfriends on my track team asked, "Becki, since you were so athletic, how can you have your leg taken away and not be angry?"

I responded, "Well, sure, I loved having two legs, but that's not the most important thing to me. If anything, my body often distracted me. Now it's easier to see that what truly matters is my relationship with God, how I'm living and who I'm loving."

Many of my friends knew I was a Christian. They also knew my dad was a pastor, which in itself was sort of a stigma. But I let my friends know that my beliefs were my own and not imposed by my dad. They knew that church and Campus Life were also important to me.

Some of my friends had ignored the spiritual side of me because they weren't Christians. After I lost my leg, they began to say, "You're different. Why aren't you reacting to your amputation like I would?"

Finally, they listened as I told them about my faith in Jesus Christ and that I was living for something much more lasting than what I was physically. "My relationship with Christ gives me a higher purpose than just what I could accomplish with my physical body," I said. "After all, I have given my life to God; it was really *his* leg that was lost, not mine."

I knew God had answered prayers for my healing. He *had* healed me—emotionally. Incredibly, I never experienced serious depression or anger over my amputation. Incredible to me and unbelievable to everyone else! Only my family and close friends knew I wasn't acting. People, from the very first day, tried to talk me into anger or tell me I was in denial. People urged me to "get in touch with my feelings." I was—and my feelings were fine!

I know this attitude was God's doing, because I know myself! I don't usually say, "O.K. Praise the Lord, and pass the potatoes!" I'm not a hokey Christian whose frothy faith glides me through any circumstance. I usually give God a fight or at least a quiz before I yield to his ultimate power and authority. This was an extraordinary reaction for me, but God never told us life with him would be ordinary.

Shortly after my surgery, I had to choose a book for an English-class report. Since I had been impressed by Joni when I met her in person, I decided to read her book. Her attitudes strongly molded the way I dealt with my disability. I remember thinking, "I can learn from her times of anger and depression so that maybe I won't go through all of that. Maybe I can skip to be where her life was at the end of the book when she could see God using her disability. I want this amputation to be something positive."

I realized my disability could by no means compare to her quadriplegia, which affects much more of life than an amputation. But I saw that her attitudes applied to my situation. Her life dramatically affected mine, especially in how she wanted to praise the Lord by everything she did.

### I Want to Do It All

Many activities were exciting achievements for me the first few weeks after surgery. I enjoyed inventing new techniques to play old favorite sports. I learned to ride a bike with one leg, roller skate with crutches and play other sports by hopping. I was a great soccer player because I had a leg plus two sticks to kick with. I could block passes with my crutches and sometimes reach out farther than other players.

When swimming, I had to utilize my arms more than before. Getting on and off the diving board with one leg was a trick, and climbing up the ladder to the high dive was a real adventure! My endurance quickly developed so that I could play volleyball for hours, hopping on one leg.

About twelve weeks after surgery I visited my sister Brenda who was working at a camp in Colorado. While there, I rode a horse for the first time after my amputation. It was strange having only one leg to hold onto the horse. The balance was different, and it seemed to throw the horse off when I tried to stand in the stirrup.

I tried about every sport. True, I couldn't do them all. Tennis was hard because I hadn't been a good tennis player with two legs. My hand–eye coordination was awful. I was always chasing the ball. Some sports, I decided, weren't practical for me. I was pleasantly surprised, however, to realize that I could do most things. It was fun to participate in sports and other activities like any other person. During this time I realized that sports could be an important bridge of hope for people with all kinds of disabilities.

## Maybe I'll Be A . . .

In my senior year of high school I met my first recreation therapist while I was learning to ski as an amputee at Winter Park, Colorado. She was my ski instructor. I began to think this would be the perfect career for me. I enjoyed people and was able to do many sports. Besides, I was academically sound in the sciences I would need for a recreation therapy degree.

My own disability would be an additional "perk" for understanding the people I'd be working with as a recreation therapist. I had learned firsthand that sports and recreation enable people to feel "normal." The handicapped person enjoys experiencing what other people do.

Athletics and recreational activities build self-confidence, as well as muscle coordination and ability. Sports can help a disabled person improve beyond the traditional progress made in therapy. It's also more fun and exciting to play a game than to work in a therapy session.

I decided this was the career God wanted me to pursue. I planned to attend a Christian college for a couple years and then transfer to a state school to finish the specific requirements of my degree.

I chose to start at Taylor University in Indiana. While I was getting used to college life, the other students were getting used to me. Many of them told me I was the first handicapped friend they had ever had. A few may have had a relative who had lost a leg in the war or because of diabetes, but most of them didn't have a one-legged peer who was going to be a part of their everyday life.

At Taylor I could be myself, educating my friends about my disability, carrying out daily activities and having fun. For the Halloween party my freshman year I went dressed as a pirate—peg leg, eye patch and all. For the peg leg, I used a bathroom plunger fastened to the end of my stump. Another time a friend kidnapped Harold the Hairless Wonder (my artificial leg) and held him for ransom. It was good to see my friends feeling comfortable with my disability.

**Positive Suffering**

Besides people like Joni, an important role model for me was Sandy. She was my roommate at Taylor and my apartment mate when we later moved to San Diego. We grew to be best friends during those years. To look at Sandy, most people would think she is a normal, healthy young woman, but Sandy wrestles with a chronic intestinal illness, Crohn's disease, which was diagnosed when she was only eight years old.

The amazing thing about Sandy is the way she lives with this debilitating ailment. Some days her abdominal pain is so bad she can't get out of bed. Many times she has to be on a complete liquid diet for weeks. Often she feels so weak she can't carry out the simplest everyday tasks.

Sandy has taught me not to use suffering as an excuse. She doesn't complain. In fact, she bears her situation very silently. Many times I have watched her quietly enduring tremendous discomfort. She isn't afraid to ask people to pray for her when she is having pain, but she doesn't seek sympathy by constantly whining, "Oh, what a terrible thing I have to live with."

When people look at me, they easily see I am disabled. They give me support and encouragement for what I am doing. When people look at Sandy, they don't see any problem. They don't realize that Sandy, and the other "Sandys" of the world with hidden illnesses, are being very heroic and courageous in the way they live.

## Without Complaining

Sandy greatly influenced my ability to handle pain when it came down to the nitty-gritty of everyday living. She prepared me for the decline in people's support after the first few months following my amputation and for the reality of living with daily discomfort.

It's one thing to go through a traumatic surgery and the terror of cancer while people applaud and say, "Good job; well done!" It's harder to wear an artificial leg every day and put up with backaches, blisters on my stump and getting fatigued sixty per cent faster than other people because of the energy it takes to propel the leg. The everyday difficulties are more trying, in some ways, than the initial loss. God used Sandy to teach me how to live the routine of life for God's glory without complaining—and to look beyond myself and my pain to other people's needs.

I can see how God used those first weeks, months and years preparing me for the ministry he would give me later on. He was getting me ready to care for other people who have illnesses and disabilities. Perhaps I have more understanding and compassion toward my patients than an able-bodied person might have. I have been there. I know what it feels like.

It's exciting to reflect on all the experiences God has given me, knowing that each one was a part of his plan, just as the Bible says, "It is God himself who has made us what we are . . . long ages ago he planned that we should spend these lives in helping others" (Eph 2:10, LB).

I am now eleven years away from the experience of losing my leg. It really did happen! But God also really did prepare me for all that was to come.

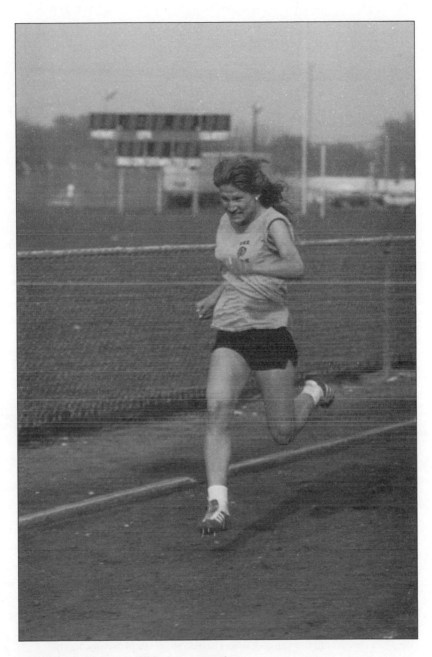

Running in a track meet before her amputation.

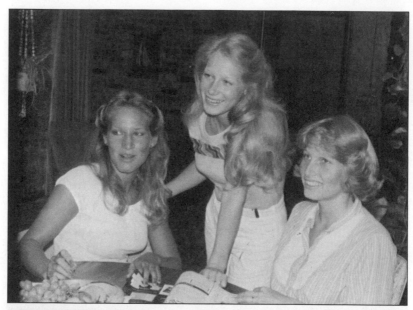

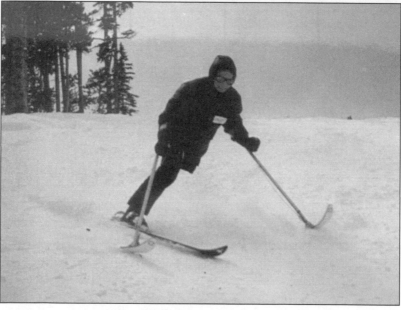

top photo: Becki (left) relaxing with sisters Brenda (center) and Barbara (right).
bottom photo: Racing down the ski slopes of Colorado.

98

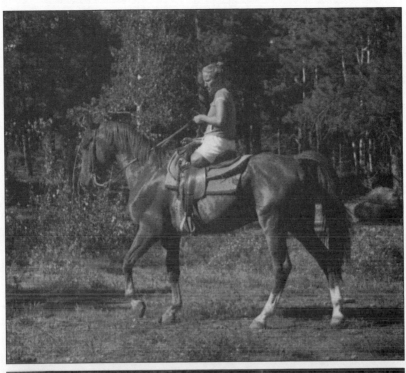

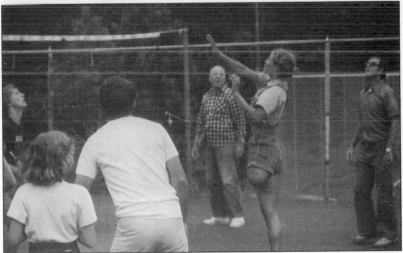

At Horn Creek Ranch in Colorado Becki enjoys horseback riding (above) and volley-ball (below).

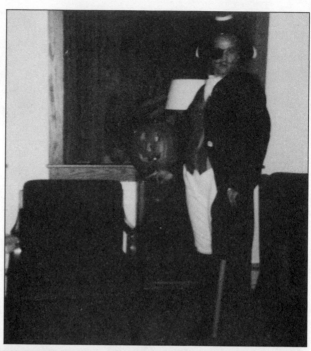

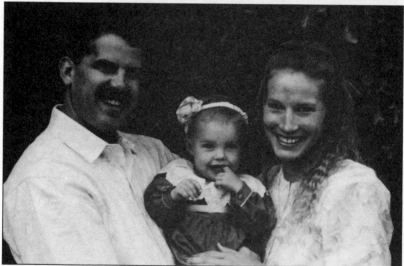

top photo: Dressed as a pegleg pirate for a college Halloween party.
bottom photo: Hayden (18 months) receives special attention from Craig and Becki.

# Part III

# GOD GIVES ASSISTANCE

# 8

## A FATHER'S PERSPECTIVE

# WORKING THROUGH A CRISIS

As I sat by myself, outside the door of the morgue in the basement of Carle Hospital, I wondered if I would ever preach again. I was glad that two years earlier our church had agreed to have the Moody Men's Chorale sing in our church on April 2, which turned out to be the Sunday after Becki's amputation. That would give me more breathing space, more time to decide if I could stay in the ministry.

A few months before Becki's surgery, however, I had accepted an invitation to speak at a midweek chapel service at Taylor University in Upland, Indiana. Our other two daughters were students at Taylor, and Becki frequently visited the campus as a high-school student. The Taylor students had been very involved in praying for Becki's healing before surgery, and they knew she had ended up losing her leg.

Over the next few days, as I thought about the invitation, I decided that I should keep this speaking engagement. It would give me an opportunity to get away from my pressure-packed situation and the nagging question "Could I stay in the ministry?" The six-hour round-trip drive alone would also be good therapy for me.

On the way to Taylor, I tried to sort out my feelings and thoughts. What did people say or do that was helping me through my crisis? What hurtful actions and attitudes could have been avoided? I decided to share with the students as honestly as I could about my experience. I wasn't going to explain or justify God's part in the situation.

I asked that the pulpit be removed from the stage and that I be given only a stool and a music stand. I just wanted to sit and chat with the students. That way, I wouldn't come across as a preacher. The result was that God greatly ministered to the students and to *me*. Speaking at the Taylor chapel helped me work through the emotional trauma of Becki's amputation and crystallized my thinking about the best way to help others in a similar situation.

At that time I had two earned master's degrees and was completing my first doctorate—all in people-helping fields. Yet, as I worked through my own crisis in the days following Becki's surgery, I learned more about helping people in crisis than in all my formal degree programs. Becki's surgery gave me a crash course in practical ways to help traumatized people.

## Experience the Body of Christ

In the midst of my crisis, I became painfully aware of the need for Christians to actively help someone work through a crisis by giving themselves in love to that person. Jesus said that the pre-eminent characteristic of love is to mark us as his disciples (Jn 13:35). Also, we are to love one another in the same sacrificial way that Jesus loves us: "Love each other *just as much* as I have loved you" (Jn 13:34 LB, emphasis mine).

Christ's command didn't mean simply greeting each other in the foyer of the church, sending Christmas cards or debating the inconsequential minutiae of theology. It meant doing whatever it took to love each other *"just as much"* as Jesus loved us.

Caring for one another is a theme repeated throughout the New Testament: "If one part [of the body] suffers, all parts suffer with it, and if one part is honored, all the parts are glad. . . . All of you together are the one body of Christ and each of you is a separate and necessary part of it" (1 Cor. 12:14-27 LB).

I realized that in any crisis one friend can't give everything that is needed to help. Each person in the body of Christ has been given abilities by God to enrich other body members. Christ provided many people who sacrificially gave to me through their prayers and physical presence.

## Build Relationships Now

It would have been unusual if a complete stranger could have provided the depth of help I needed in the middle of my intense crisis. The foundation of trust just wouldn't have been there. Friends who already knew me well were the greatest source of help.

Three friends were a tremendous help to me immediately after Becki's amputation. As I sat outside the door to the morgue, I felt totally alone. I was sure that my closest friend, God, had abandoned me. What would I do now? Suddenly I felt a hand on my shoulder. I turned around to see Dick, the senior pastor of another church in town. We had served together in many different ministries in the community. We often met privately to share our joys and woes in ministry. We jokingly talked about trading some of our most difficult people to each other. We had a solid friendship.

Dick smiled gently and said to me, "Conway, I've checked on Becki in the recovery room. She's going to make it, but I'm worried about you. Thousands of people in this community are watching how you'll react to this whole crisis. I want you to know I care for you." Dick didn't say much more, but his presence gave me stability when my foundation—God—seemed gone.

Two other men came to me in those early days, almost in rotation. One man, Jim, was the chairman of our church board and also the Campus Life director. The third man, Brock, was on our pastoral staff. One at a time they sat with me in a small, private room in the hospital.

I had known these men for many years. I trusted them and believed they cared for me. I could say anything to these men. I knew my problem with God wouldn't destroy our friendship or undermine their faith in God. So I unloaded on them: "Where was God when Becki was having her leg cut off? I'll bet he was so busy answering somebody's prayer to find a parking place that he didn't have time to heal Becki's leg!"

I asked them, "How can I possibly go back into the pulpit and teach the Bible as true? How can I say that prayer works? After all, I wasn't the one who dreamed up the idea of praying. It was God who said, 'Ask and you will receive' (Mt 7:7). Jesus promised, 'If two of you on earth agree about anything you ask for, it will be done for you by my Father in heaven' (Mt 18:19). *Jesus* is the one who said, 'If you have faith as small as a mustard seed, you can say to this mountain, "Move. . . ." Nothing will be impossible for you' (Mt 17:20)."

I continued dumping on these friends. "It was God who urged us to bring our petitions before him. *I* didn't come to God and say, 'Hey God, I've thought of this neat idea. I'll bring my concerns to you, I'll ask for your blessing and help; then you will have an opportunity to demonstrate your power.' No, prayer was all God's idea, and now he has led me out onto the end of a branch and sawed the branch off!"

I poured out my feelings of disillusionment, my uncertainty about the future, my anguish for Becki. After all, I had promised Becki that her leg wouldn't come off. How would I face her? How could I face all the other Christians who had heard me preach and who had watched prayer work in so many other instances?

It took a special kind of person, one who had a deep relationship with me, to be able to walk into that dim corridor outside the morgue and lift me out of my pit of despair. It took friends who knew and accepted me to sit in that little hospital conference room and listen to me rail in rage at God.

In the days after that experience, when I was able to see beyond my own needs, I could ask myself, "Who am I building relationships with that are deep enough so I can help them when *they* struggle with hard questions?" I was grateful I could pour out my heart to friends who didn't flinch and who loved me through my pain. I was glad I hadn't waited until I was in crisis to start those friendships. In the middle of my crisis, I had nothing to give to build a mutual relationship.

## Comfort Out Of Pain

In times of pain, we naturally look for "comfort passages" in Scripture. One section, especially, gave me a broader under–

standing of the pain and comfort concept:

> What a wonderful God we have—he is the father of our Lord Jesus Christ, the source of every mercy, the one who so wonderfully comforts and strengthens us in our hardships and trials. And why does he do this? So that when others are troubled, needing our sympathy and encouragement, we can pass on to them this same help and comfort God has given us (2 Cor 1:3-4 LB).

This passage presupposes I will experience pain and problems. Only after I accept trials as normal, can I receive God's promise of comfort. His expectation then is that I use his comfort and encouragement to bless another hurting person. If I don't suffer, I won't have anything to offer to others. My pain becomes a bridge into another struggler's life.

Yet, in spite of all I've learned, when I'm in the midst of a difficult situation, my first prayer usually is, "God, if you love me, get me out of this problem. I don't want any more pain or suffering." God, however, tells me he is going to use my pain and crises to transform me into a more sensitive, caring person with something to offer another person.

Before Becki's surgery, I was in mid-life crisis for over a year and was extremely depressed. I wasn't functioning well as a husband or father or senior pastor of a large church. During this extremely difficult year, Sally and I had been doing research about men who were experiencing mid-life crisis. I had signed a contract a year earlier to write a book which was due in six weeks. I had not written one word. The project appeared to be as difficult as scaling Mt. Everest.

I was sitting at my makeshift desk in the basement of our Urbana home, pouring out my heart to God. "Lord, why do I have to go through this mid-life crisis? Why do I have to experience this terrible depression? Why do I have to feel so unfulfilled at my job, and why must I experience this terrible sense of failure as a father and husband?"

After I had poured out my heart to God for several minutes, God reminded me of 2 Corinthians 1:3-4. I sensed God saying to me, "Your pain, Jim, will give you the ability to write, to counsel, to offer help to men and women who are experiencing what you are experiencing. You will become believable because you have been there. Allow me to bring healing to other people through your pain."

I sat there for a long time, reflecting on my dialog with God. Finally, I said, "I want you to use me, Lord. I want to help people. If pain will give me the ability to help more effectively, then I'm willing for pain to happen. I only ask that you comfort me in the depth of my being as I go through this pain."

People all around me were in pain because of sickness, death, poverty, loss of jobs, broken marriages, broken relationships and failures of every sort. How could they possibly identify with me if I had never experienced hurt or loss? How could my message be believed if I was viewed as a creature from another planet? I decided I wouldn't hide my pain. I would let the fact of my pain and the gracious comfort I've received from God be the loving gift that I would offer to a hurting friend.

## Let Grief Spill Out

Another truth I experienced firsthand during Becki's ordeal was the important role that grief plays in the healing process. Trying to stop me from expressing grief and sorrow would have been useless. My grief would have bubbled up in some form. Holding grief down is like trying to hold two dozen Ping-Pong balls under the water at the same time. They keep slipping out from under our hands and bobbing to the surface.

Suppressed grief can threaten emotional and spiritual health and becomes a festering sore that will express itself some way sooner or later. Discouraging people from expressing grief communicates either that their grief is wrong or that we don't care.

A young woman named Joanne had been sexually molested by her father from the time she was eight years old into her mid-teen years. The repeated experience horrified her. She tried to compensate by totally erasing thoughts of her father from her mind. No one was sensitive enough to give her the opportunity to pour out her grief and bitterness. So the pent-up grief and anger came out in the form of physically abusing herself. She pounded her body so that she had ugly black-and-blue marks all over and also went on life-threatening starvation diets. In addition, she started running around with a wild bunch of young men who sexually exploited her.

When I got to know Joanne, I realized this woman didn't need someone to tell her to stop beating her body, eat normally and quit her sexual involvements. She needed someone to listen, to let the torrents of bitterness and anger pour out. She needed someone just "to be with her" as she relived the horrible experiences of her past. Once she was allowed to express her pain, her life started to stabilize and the self-destructive patterns disappeared.

Expressing our problems is similar to what happens in an earthquake. When a large amount of pressure builds up and the earth is forced to make a large adjustment, great damage occurs to property and lives. However, if the earth makes small shifts frequently, pressure is relieved gradually and little damage occurs.

The same is true if we share about troubles as they come along. Like a small earth tremor, no great damage occurs. But disregarding small struggles causes them to build up. When we finally open up, a horrendous explosion may take place that causes great damage to everyone.

For these reasons, I try not to restrain another person's grief.

I am cautious about saying, "All things work together for good. Don't be discouraged. Things are bound to get better."

If I were to say things like that, I might actually mean, "Please be quiet. Your pain disturbs me too much."

It's not hard to imitate Job's friends. His so-called comforters frequently tried to stop him from sharing how he really felt. They believed his words were an attack on God. It was as if they were saying to Job, "Hush. Shhhh. Don't say any more. God will hear you."

God is a big boy. He can take anything that we dish out. His self-image is never going to be damaged by our questions. We don't have to protect God. In fact, he will stay with us through our questioning times and still love us unconditionally.

When my friends are pouring out their grief, I try to let them dump out all their ugly feelings. My role as a true, loving comforter is just to listen. My best help is just being there. I must set aside my need to feel good as a "helper" with solutions and just concentrate on listening to my friend's feelings. It's probably enough for me to say, "I'm your friend and I want to be with you as you walk through this terrible time."

**No Easy Answers, Please**

A further truth that came through loud and clear after Becki's amputation was the damaging effect of glib answers. Several people tried to help me by explaining why things had turned out as they had. I have mentioned one man who thought the purpose for Becki's surgery was to bring revival to the church. I am sure people's intentions were good. But their answers drove me even deeper into despair, causing me to be angry at them for their misguided, inane answers.

One day I was standing in the hall outside Becki's hospital room because I needed to be alone. I just couldn't handle the sight of Becki's loss and the reality that my prayer was not answered. I needed a moment of solitude to regain my composure.

While I stood in a quiet part of the hallway, a man came alongside and said, "Jim, I think I know why Becki's amputation has happened." I had heard these words so often that I immediately put up my defenses, hoping not to be hurt again by another well-meaning person who thought he had to have an answer.

But I was totally unprepared for this man's answer to the problem. He said, "For a number of years I've listened to you preach. I really believe you speak too much about the 'love of God.' I think God has allowed this to happen so that you will begin to preach more about the 'justice' and 'holiness' of God."

It was all I could do to keep my right arm down at my side. I had a deep, raging desire to double my fist and punch his teeth into his stomach. What kind of God did this man worship—a fiendish God who delights in maiming people and then, if they can't understand why things happen, he laughs and knocks them down?

My heart was pounding in my throat. My eyes were flaming. With all the control I could muster, I turned and walked further away down the quiet hallway. The hurt that he had inflicted on me was so great that it was almost unbearable. On top of the feeling that God had abandoned me by allowing Becki's leg to be amputated, I now had this new anger and pain.

The attempted answers of this man, and others like him, only increased the intensity of my hurt. Their puny answers were a distortion of the person of God and an insult to my beautiful sixteen-year-old daughter.

**Someday . . .**
I have learned to face the reality that many questions in life will not be answered until we step into eternity. Life is full of am-

biguity and paradox. There isn't a neat Bible verse for every situation in life. In my life, Becki's amputation is one of these unanswered questions.

The Bible tells us, "We can see and understand only a little about God now, as if we were peering at His reflection in a poor mirror" (1 Cor 13:12 LB).

We finite human beings will never in this life fully understand an infinite God. Only when we reach heaven will we know God's purposes more completely. Looking for reasons for every problem isn't always productive. I've learned that life can go on even though we may not know all of the explanations for our pain. God will be present in the midst of my swirling storm of unanswered questions. We can continue talking to God even in our confusion.

God isn't going to lift us out of the pressures of life, but he does promise to be with us. He often has steadied me with these assurances:

When they walk through the Valley of Weeping it will become a place of springs where pools of blessing and refreshment collect after rains! They will grow constantly in strength and each of them is invited to meet with the Lord. . . . For Jehovah God is our Light and our Protector. (Ps 84:6–7, 11 LB)

# 9

## A FATHER'S PERSPECTIVE

# LET GOD
# BE GOD

*I was in my study preparing messages for the coming* Sunday when I received a desperate phone call. Peggy was almost hysterical as she said, "Pastor, please come quickly!" Her next-door neighbors were fighting, and she was hearing horrible screams. "I'll be right over," I told her.

I put on my suit coat, grabbed my Bible and ran to the car. Peggy lived only a few blocks away, but in those few minutes all kinds of thoughts rushed through my head. I wondered what was happening in that house next door. How could I calm the situation? Would I be able to help this young couple resolve their problems? I hoped I'd be able to share with them how much God loved them. Perhaps I could even get them started coming regularly to church.

I was a young pastor, fresh out of seminary, and I felt that God had given me a mandate to win the world for Jesus. Certainly God was going to use this event as a spiritual blessing in the lives of this young couple.

I tore into Peggy's driveway, screeched to a halt and jumped out of the car. I asked Peggy what was happening now. She said she wasn't sure. She had heard a lot of fighting all morning. Then came those awful screams. Since she'd called me, it had been deathly silent.

## The Terrifying Silence

Because I was a "take charge" young pastor, I walked over to the side door and knocked on the screen door. "Is anybody home? I'd like to talk to you. My name is Pastor Conway. I'd be glad to help if I can."

There was only silence from inside the house. The door inside the screen door was open about halfway. I opened the screen door and went into the house onto a small landing. Several steps to my left led down to the basement. Three more steps to my right led up into the kitchen.

I repeatedly called out, "Hello. Is anyone home? My name is Pastor Conway. I'd like to help. Is anyone home?" Still no response came from anyone inside the house.

As I spoke, I inched my way up the three steps into the kitchen. I could see the remains of breakfast on the kitchen table. The kitchen counter was also cluttered. Things were scattered around the floor where they shouldn't have been. Obviously, something was wrong. I could feel danger.

The kitchen was L-shaped. From my vantage point, I

couldn't see the entire kitchen. I continued to ask, "Is anyone home? I am Pastor Conway. I'd like to help if I can." Slowly I advanced farther into the kitchen.

Then I saw her! The young woman was lying on the kitchen floor. She was motionless. Blood was splattered on the upper part of her body. It looked as if she had been stabbed repeatedly.

My first thought was, "Oh, dear God, she's dead!" And then I realized that she was a full-term pregnant woman. I wondered if the baby were still alive. What was I going to do now? Her husband obviously had stabbed her. I could feel his presence. Was he in the basement? Would he have blocked off my escape from the house? Or was he just around the corner in the dining room?

Terror gripped my throat, and I realized that I was in way over my head. I quickly beat a retreat out the side door and told Peggy, "Call the police. It looks as if the wife has been stabbed to death."

## Surround the House

Peggy rushed into her house, called the police and gave them what information we had. I stood outside the house, wondering how we could get the young woman's body out and perhaps save the baby.

It seemed like hours, but in reality, it was only minutes before the police arrived. They quickly surrounded the house. The sergeant asked me in detail about what I had seen and if I knew whether the man was armed with more than a knife.

After the police had thoroughly surveyed the situation, an officer began calling out to the young husband inside, "Your house is totally surrounded by the police. You cannot escape. Put your weapons down and come outside. Give yourself up." They repeated the command a number of times during the next several minutes.

By this time, the neighbors in this little town of fifteen thousand had gathered around the entire perimeter of the young couple's fenced backyard. The word had spread quickly. Murder is not a common occurrence in a farming community. Cars began to clog the street, with little access left for the ambulance.

## The Assault

The police finally decided to rush the house and try to save the baby in the dead mother. The front door was locked, so they chose to kick in the door. At a predetermined moment, two officers rushed the front door while two rushed the side door. As they broke through the front door into the living room, the young husband jumped through a rear bedroom window and started running wildly across the yard. He still carried the knife which he had used to kill his wife.

The drama was unbelievable. Neighbors totally surrounded the backyard fence. The young husband was running across the backyard with the knife in his hand. Two policeman drew a bead on the running man, and three shots rang out. The young man crumpled to the ground. I was amazed that no bystander was hit by the bullets.

The police rushed to the wounded man. He was quickly put on a stretcher and carried to the ambulance. Other ambulance attendants were now carrying the body of the young woman to the same ambulance.

Hours before, the couple had been fighting with each other. Now they would ride in the same ambulance—one of them dead, the other seriously wounded and their unborn child's fate unknown.

Why had this happened? Why had this young husband lost all hope? What had caused him to sink so deeply into a pit of despair that he had finally killed his wife?

It was weeks before some of the questions were answered. The man was a student, frustrated by mounting bills. His wife would not be able to work after the baby came, and he felt inadequate to care for his family. In addition, he was studying psychology, which was highly suspect by his family and the people in his home church. Some folks in his home community even thought that psychology was demonic.

In the middle of his crisis, with little family and community support and mounting financial pressure, he felt trapped. He and his wife fought often. Another verbal conflict had broken out that morning at breakfast. It got worse. He began shoving and hitting. Finally he crossed over the line of self-control and repeatedly stabbed his wife until she bled to death. Their un-born baby also died.

## God or Ultimate Despair

In my years as a pastor I have often seen that a terrible ca-lamity or problem either moves people toward God by trusting him with the uncertain future or moves them toward despair. I came to this place following Becki's amputation and found there is no middle ground. The crisis eliminated the luxury of compromise and forced me to some kind of immediate action. The ultimate choice became: trust God or trust myself. If I chose not to trust God, ultimately I would be choosing despair.

The basic question I wrestled with was: "Will I let God be God? Will I let him do this to me? Or will I make every effort to take charge of this situation because I feel I cannot trust God?"

The situation seemed unfair. It was unreasonable that God allowed Becki's amputation to happen. I decided I had to trust myself since God had let me down. It was terribly lonely just trusting myself. During that time of not trusting God, I was forced to rethink my views about God, prayer, life's problems and my relationship with other Christians. I got down to some gut-level insights.

I wasn't afraid to question. I realized the only thing I had to fear was isolating myself from God. I knew I had to keep talking to him about my questions. Ultimately, I chose to surrender to God, deciding that he loves my family and wants the very best for us.

## God Isn't the Same as Christians

Frequently, we don't allow God to be God in our lives because we think he is the same as some Christians who are poor imitations of Jesus. When we have a problem, some Christians around us imply that they alone have "the truth."

Ralph was one of these well-intentioned Christians. One day he asked, "Now, Pastor, I don't want to pry, but is your family really praying and believing God for a miracle? Are you praying in Jesus' name and claiming the victory he accomplished on the cross?" Ralph was a "name-it-and-claim-it" Christian. He felt that God was obligated to do anything he directed him to do. He reasoned that if our prayers weren't being answered, we must not be praying correctly.

Some mistaken people believe that no Christian should ever suffer. Many of them believe that God intends to heal every Christian who asks. They cannot accept the book of Job at face value—that God really allowed Job to experience all of those calamities. Or they side with Job's comforters, suggesting that something was wrong with Job that is not written in the account.

These people do not believe that Paul was actually given a thorn in the flesh. They have a simplistic view of the Scriptures which causes them to see God only as a "Sugar Daddy" who would never allow us to experience pain, sickness, unhappi-

ness or poverty. Because these Christians have a limited understanding of Scripture, they tend to try to make people with
problems feel guilty.

My disappointment with God made me more vulnerable to
this type of Christian and tempted me to move away from God.
It's a terrible feeling to be with Christians and yet be so
wounded by them. We naturally want to get away from the
people who cause the pain.

During this time of deep stress, the only way I could handle
Christians such as Ralph was to say to myself, "These people
are well-intentioned, but they are missing the full meaning of
the Scriptures." It was important for me not to assume that
God was the same as Ralph. God was not going to make me
jump through special hoops. He knew the cry of my heart and
the urgent prayer request from our family and church. I had to
be careful not to run from God in my attempt to escape the
harassment of misinformed Christians.

## Back to the Basics about God

My ability to "let God be God" came from reaffirming some
basic concepts from the Scripture about who God really is.
After my initial anger at God, I constantly reminded myself that
*God* will always be God. *Even if I chose not to allow him
to be God* in my life, that wouldn't change the reality that he
will always be the God of everything. He will not give up his
position, no matter what happens. Neither will God be manip-
ulated by my prayers or any circumstances in my life.

I also had to admit that a certain degree of *mystery* will
always be attached to God. God is infinite, endless, unlimited.
I, on the other hand, am finite and limited. Only after I step into
eternity will I begin to know more about God.

Then, I had to concede that God has *infinite insight*. God
was present before the world began. He'll exist after it ends. He

knows everything that's going to happen before it happens. He knew my family before the world was created. He knows everything about us. He has absolutely correct insight into what is best for us.

At the time of Becki's surgery, when I asked, "Shall I let God be God?" I realized that no one else in the universe knows more about me and what is best for me than God. To limit the decisions for my future to my pygmy experience and background would be extreme foolishness.

I also admitted that God is *holy*. God is absolutely pure, without one wrong thought or motive. He is absolutely correct about my situation. God will not make a mistake.

Thinking of God's holiness reminded me of his *love*. God is the father who sent his only Son into the world to die as a sacrifice on the cross for me. He is the mother hen who gathers me under her wings for protection. God's love for me is constant, even though I yell in his face or impune his motives.

God would never say to me, "Oops! I made a mistake. I led you down the wrong trail." Neither is he going to say, "Ha, ha! You thought I loved you. What I really meant to say was, 'I'll love you only if you do good stuff and never sin.' "

I consciously reminded myself that God's love is *unconditional.* The Bible says:

> If his children forsake my laws and don't obey them, then I will punish them, but I will never completely take away my loving kindness from them, nor let my promise fail. No, I will not break my covenant; I will not take back one word of what I said." (Ps 89:30–34, LB)

I knew that God's love for me would continue forever. He might punish me if I do wrong, but the correction would be only for the purpose of bringing me back to him. I wish I could report to you that I no longer need his correction nor do I have struggles with various sins. Unfortunately, that's not the case.

I also saw God's love for me as *redemptive*. My crisis was an opportunity for God to show me his love and kindness by bringing good out of the situation. God plans good for *me* and my family—he will not exploit us! Christians have exploited me, let me down, put guilt trips on me, ignored me or avoided me—but not God! As I thought about the basics of who God really is, it was easier to "let God be God."

## A New View of Prayer

As I admitted who God really was, my view of prayer was altered. I realized that prayer would never put me in charge of God. God is not a genie in the bottle who pops out to do my bidding when I rub the prayer bottle. God will always retain his sovereignty and will always reserve the right to answer my prayer with a clear, "No."

Then what should prayer be, if I can't get what I ask for? Prayer is intended to *help me acknowledge my need*. It is a way to admit that I am not self-sufficient, to admit to God and myself that I am not a "god" and to acknowledge that I need God's leadership in my life.

This truth, which was vividly reinforced at Becki's amputation, has carried me through some later difficulties. A few years ago Sally and I accepted a call to teach at Talbot Seminary, part of Biola University in La Mirada, California. We firmly believed this was God's call, yet it was going to create a tremendous hardship because of the high cost of housing in that area. Our combined salaries would not cover the cost of our home mortgage.

Before we moved, I had a recurring dream. We were in California and unable to pay our bills. Even though we had sold all our personal possessions, we ended up bankrupt and without a place to live. I would wake up in a cold sweat every night.

After we moved, Sally and I had to repeatedly admit to God

that we could not handle this financial strain. We needed his provision; he was our only resource. And God was sufficient. Month after month he miraculously provided what we needed to live in California.

In the weeks after Becki's operation, I had to admit that prayer is not coming to some giant celestial smorgasbord where I can pick up any goodie I would like. Rather, prayer is my *agreement with God,* an acknowledgment of who he is and consenting to his purpose in my life, whatever that is. He wants me to grant him the right to be God, telling him that I am willing to allow growth to come through pain and problems.

## A New View of Stress and Problems

It's easier for me to permit "God to be God" if I think of problems as the messengers of God for my growth. That's easy to say, but it's never been easy for me to do. When Becki lost her leg, I didn't see this as God's message for my growth. I recoiled in anger and frustration. I've told you before that my initial reaction to problems is usually, "God, if you love me, get me out of this mess!"

God's answer, however, was, "Because I love you, I'm keeping you in this problem." God has this great knack of looking farther than I look. He's able to see beyond the problem to what will be accomplished because of the problem. I had to stick with God even though I didn't completely trust him. That process took time, but God also understood that.

The following words from the Bible have seemed unsettling or encouraging, depending on my circumstances:

Dear brothers, is your life full of difficulties and temptations? Then be happy, for when the way is rough, your patience has a chance to grow. So let it grow, and don't try to squirm out of your problems. For when your patience is finally in full bloom, then you will be ready for anything, strong in character, full and complete. (Jas 1:2-4, LB)

The teaching in these verses is that problems are not my enemies; they are my friends that help me develop patience and maturity. Problems don't catch God off guard. Problems are a normal part of life which God uses for my development.

When I measured myself against these verses, I realized that if I were to be living a biblical life, I should "be happy" when a problem or crisis comes. I'm not supposed to be exuberant because of the problem itself, but because of what the problem accomplishes in my life. I don't say, "God, I thank you that my daughter had her leg chopped off because of cancer." But ultimately I have come to say, "God, by faith I thank you for the end product of this tragedy—that we will all grow and mature because of this crisis."

## The Hard Freeze

I appreciate the story about a young man in Texas who bought land and began to grow orange trees. The man became very prosperous, bought more land and planted more trees. He was very careful to give God a part of his earnings.

One very cold winter the orange trees were severely damaged because of a very hard freeze. They had to be cut off about a foot above the ground and rebudded. He would not have a fruit crop for another five years—a financial disaster.

The man became very angry at God. He stopped going to church, quit reading his Bible and totally withdrew from all Christians.

After a year or so, a new pastor came to the local church. He was an older man who had lived a lot of life and had shared much grief with the people he had pastored. He visited the bitter orange-grower and asked if he could help. The old pastor sat there while the younger man poured out his anger and bitter venom against God. "Why would God do this to me? If he's as smart as he says he is, he knows that orange trees can't stand a hard freeze. Why did he let the hard freeze come?"

The older pastor listened patiently. When the tirade quieted down, he said to the younger man, "Yes, God knows that orange trees can't grow with a hard freeze. But God also knows that men can't grow *without* a hard freeze."

## Why Did Christ Stay on the Cross?

I mentioned earlier that after Becki's surgery I was to speak at Taylor University. I had more than three hours to meditate as I drove by myself to the campus. During that time God reminded me of a picture given to me as a college student. It showed Jesus hanging on the cross. Dark, angry clouds filled the background.

I thought about Christ in the garden before he was taken to Golgotha to die. He had prayed, "Not my will, but yours be done." Then I thought of Christ on the cross. People taunted him, "If you are God as you say you are, then come down from the cross."

"Why didn't Christ choose *his* will in the garden instead of the will of the Godhead?" I asked myself. "Why did Christ stay on the cross and die, instead of coming down and demonstrating his power as he could have?"

Of course, I had known the answer all along. Christ deliberately stayed on the cross, because he had a higher purpose of providing payment for our sins.

It wasn't that the Father was unable to take Christ off the cross. Instead, by deliberate choice of the Godhead, Christ stayed on the cross.

## In the Operating Room

Then my thoughts flashed to Becki's operating room. Even

though I had never seen the place, I saw it then in my mind. Becki was stretched out on that cold table. Doctors and nurses were gathered around her. God was there, too. His hands were gently on her shoulders. He was patting her as if to calm her and to keep her on the operating table. He was saying to her and to me, "It's all right, my child. I have a higher purpose in mind."

I saw the point so clearly then! God was not incapable of taking Christ off the cross or Becki off the operating table. Instead he had a different purpose.

Now I had a choice to make. What would I do with God's decision? Would I allow God to be God or would I say that he was wrong? Would I install myself as God, and then end up only in terrible, frantic despair? In those moments as I drove the car toward Taylor, I deliberately chose to let God be God once more.

## We All Need Healing

Recently I spoke to about 450 men at a retreat. I felt urged by God to share about Becki, including my reactions to her amputation and what I learned from that process. Then I asked them if they had a problem or a crisis in which they needed deliberately to allow God to be God. All over the auditorium men began crying. I asked them to pray silently, giving God the right to be God in their lives.

After the period of silent prayer, I asked the men who had yielded some part of their life to God to raise a hand to seal this decision. I was astounded as I looked around the auditorium. Almost every man had raised his hand.

Then it hit me. All of us are experiencing crises. Each of us has problems. We all are being faced continually with the question, "Will I let God be God in my life or will I choose my own way? Will I be God or will I trust him to work out what's best for me?"

My feelings pushed me to not trust God. But my previous experiences with him and with Scripture encouraged me to trust him and look for good out of this crisis.

For because of our faith, He has brought us into this place of highest privilege where we now stand, and we confidently and joyfully look forward to actually becoming all that God has had in mind for us to be. We can rejoice, too, when we run into problems and trials for we know that they are good for us—they help us learn to be patient. And patience develops strength of character in us and helps us trust God more each time we use it until finally our hope and faith are strong and steady. Then, when that happens, we are able to hold our heads high no matter what happens and know that all is well, for we know how dearly God loves us, and we feel this warm love everywhere within us because God has given us the Holy Spirit to fill our hearts with His love. (Rom 5:2-5, LB)

Even as I write this chapter, my only peace about Becki's amputation comes as I repeatedly say, "O.K., God, I don't understand it, but I trust you to care for all of us. I'll let you be God."

# 10

## A MOTHER'S PERSPECTIVE

# GOD DOESN'T MAKE MISTAKES

One time, *after Becki's amputation, she and I were* shopping for clothes. We soon noticed a boy about four years old crawling under the rack of girls' skirts, trying to get a better look at Becki. He was obviously trying to figure out where her other leg was. His mother saw him and snatched him from under the rack.

"What's wrong with that girl?" he asked in a loud voice.

"Shhh!" his mother whispered. "She has no leg." The mother tried to drag the little boy farther away and to keep him quiet, but he was not to be put off.

He ran over to Becki and asked, "How'd you get your *no leg?*"

The mother was embarrassed, but Becki smiled and explained to the boy that her leg had been sick and the doctors took it off so that the rest of her body wouldn't get sick. The boy seemed to understand but continued to stare as his mother pulled him out of the store.

This "sick-leg" explanation usually satisfies most young children, but one little boy didn't let her answer end there. Becki and I were running together at the indoor track. (Becki did about two laps on one leg to my one lap on two legs!) We had stopped to rest when a little boy asked how she had lost her leg.

After she told him about her leg getting sick, he declared, "But that will never happen to me."

Becki started to say, "No, probably not . . . ," when he interrupted, " 'Cause I eat apples. Apples keep me from getting sick.' "

Then he turned and looked at Becki sternly, "Do you eat apples?"

"I do now!" she replied.

Another time Becki was roller-skating. She had been skating with a partner, so she wasn't using her crutches. As the music ended, she came rolling off the floor on just her one leg.

A little boy caught sight of her for the first time and exclaimed, "You've lost your leg!"

"I did? Oh, dear!" Becki responded in a fake surprise. She looked anxiously around her. "I'm always losing things. My mother is going to kill me for this. Will you help me hunt for my leg?"

The little boy very earnestly started looking for Becki's other leg. She eventually led him to her crutches and explained about her missing leg.

## God's Preparation

Becki's sense of humor has helped me to more concretely trust God with the realities of her amputation; however, as a mother, I want to level with you. I still agonize that Becki has to go through life without her leg. I wish she didn't have to endure the tremendous pain caused by her prosthesis. I shudder as I think of a possible time when she could be saved from danger if only she could run. I worry about her good leg deteriorating because of the extra stress it bears (other amputees have had this problem). I don't like to see a curvature developing in her spine, which causes back pain. I still have not found completely reasonable answers to why God allowed Becki's loss— *but I know God doesn't make mistakes!*

I have experienced God's hand at work in profound ways, and I know his preparation had been underway for years. After Becki's surgery I could see why God had given her that witty, spunky personality she had displayed as a little girl. Sometimes we had tried to put a damper on her because we were afraid others would think she was out of place. But God knew why he was forming her that way!

She had always been very open and forthright. With Becki, "what you saw was what you got." Whatever she was thinking usually just bubbled out. But along with her openness, she also possessed good insights and a maturing wisdom.

These qualities of insight and openness put people at ease about her missing leg. She is able to start casual conversations with new people in a way that helps them feel comfortable. They soon feel free to share with her, not just about disabilities but also about other interests. Without high pressure or contrivance, Becki often goes on to talk about her relationship with the Lord.

God also had prepared Becki for her amputation in physical ways. She, along with her sisters, was very bouncy and athletic.

*131*

In addition to sports and games, our daughters also took piano lessons—with varying success. As each girl got older and busier with other interests, she would pressure us to let her quit piano lessons.

Becki had started piano enthusiastically, but after a few years, she begged to stop. She wanted to take gymnastic lessons, but we couldn't afford those along with piano lessons. We reasoned that knowing music would be of much more value than gymnastics when she grew up.

Then a series of events brought the piano lessons to an end and Becki got her gymnastic lessons. She later was a junior-high cheerleader, as well as a hurdler on the high-school track team. All of these activities developed her physical coordination and stamina.

When I saw how quickly Becki got back to normal after her amputation, I understood why God had provided physical training for her. Immediately she could stand unwaveringly on her remaining leg. She had endurance to walk long distances on crutches or to play volleyball for hours at a time, balancing and hopping on one leg.

## God's Wise Provisions

Before Becki's surgery I sometimes wondered what life might hold for her afterwards. I knew God didn't make any mistakes, but—would she ever marry? She had several boyfriends before her amputation, but would any of them date her afterwards? Would any man want a woman without a leg?

As usual, God was way ahead of me. One of his provisions was John, a member of the high-school swim team. John and Becki had just started to date at the time we learned that Becki would have her leg removed. In their times together, he let her talk out her feelings about her upcoming surgery.

Before she entered the hospital, John told her to plan for a date as soon as she could go out after she got home. That gave her something to look forward to after surgery. Immediately after the operation he spent many hours by her bedside, helping her through the first painful part of the recovery.

As we got to know more about John, we learned that he had grown up with a "disability." He had worn leg braces for years because of a congenital hip problem. Friends told us that even with braces he participated in sports and lived a normal life. He did well in school and was liked by people of all ages. He no longer wore braces, but he knew the inconveniences of being handicapped. God used him and his understanding to help Becki—and me—at an important time.

Not only did Becki continue to have many dates over the next years, but God had a special provision in mind: Craig, whom she met at just the right time and later married. He is a very intelligent, talented and sensitive person. He is also experienced with disabled people because of his outdoor recreation work. Becki's missing leg was no big deal to him. The focus of their developing relationship was broader than her one-leggedness.

## Our Friends

Becki's friends were strategic to her recovery, and friends helped in *our* recovery too. Church members provided meals and all kinds of loving care to us. Some relatives came from other states to be with us while Becki was in the hospital. Other loved ones called us often.

One friend, Gary, a doctor of physical therapy, telephoned from out of state and gave us very important guidance about features to watch for as Becki's prosthesis was created. This was totally unmapped territory for us, and we appreciated tips from an expert.

People took time to write letters to Becki and to us. One

friend, Norma, who had undergone a radical mastectomy wrote Becki a very thoughtful letter, part of which said:

I remember the first time I ever saw you. Your folks had been camping on vacation and stopped to see us. You were just beginning to walk and were staggering around every-where. . . .

Becky, you are a beautiful girl and vibrant, and nothing will change that. As you probably know, I too have cancer . . . and I have a little inkling of what you are going through. Somehow losing part of your body is quite different than just plain surgery. I was never any Farrah Fawcett, but somehow I had gotten used to all of my body after forty-six years and sorta wanted to keep it that way!

This is not an easy thing to accept, particularly for you since your loss will be more evident than mine. However, every night and morning I look at myself and think "ugly, ugly, ugly." Yet the Lord does give grace to accept yourself and to accept His will *even* in these things.

Becky, I have the feeling you're going to bounce back from this with real victory and vitality. That's my prayer. I love you.

Norma

The cancer eventually overtook Norma, but her words were an important part in God's equipping us for our crisis. The letter greatly warmed our hearts the day it arrived, and her insights were a part of us as we went through the surgery and recovery. Her generous act of taking time to write to a sixteen-year-old at that critical moment has often been a reminder to me to take time to help someone else.

## God Creates Positive out of Negative

Along with the many helpful deeds and words of friends, a few *unhelpful* remarks were made to me following Becki's surgery, as they were to Jim, Becki and her sisters. Some people, in trying to find a reason for God not healing Becki, suggested that we did not have enough faith for God to act. I kept thinking of the grain of mustard seed that Jesus talked about, and I knew I had exercised at least *that* much faith.

One woman probably didn't realize how cruel she was as she drew me aside and asked, "Do you suppose that God didn't heal Becki because she or someone else in your family has been involved in witchcraft?"

Those words stung! Especially since that woman had been with us in the special church prayer times and had heard our family's prayers of confession and petition.

I didn't have complete answers for those people, and I still don't. Their comments had at least one positive result, however. They caused me to carefully ponder the theology of suffering.

I have seen that the Bible gives many examples of godly people who weren't healed or delivered from trials. Some of those saints, such as Job, saw their loss replaced with more than they had originally (Job 42:10-16). Paul came to accept God's purpose in allowing his physical affliction to persist (2 Cor 12:7-10). But others never did live to see a purpose for their suffering (for example, Stephen, Acts 7:54-60, and the saints listed in Hebrews 11:36-38). Even though I don't have answers, I'm sure God is not making any mistakes.

### Fake Is Always Fake

One of the most awful times for me during Becki's recovery was the day we first went to the prosthetist. It didn't help any that the day was dark and dismal. The workshop seemed gloomy and cluttered. I was appalled at the pieces of artificial limbs on counter tops, hanging from hooks and leaning here and there. They looked so grotesque and, well, fake.

As the kind prosthetist talked to us, I began to get a dreadful sense that we had been horribly misled by well-meaning people. Becki wasn't going to be running and jumping on this new leg. It wasn't going to look just like her real one. Becki would need hours of training and endure much pain to even use the thing. It would be extremely expensive ($2,000 in 1978; over $16,000 for her latest one). Because of the hard use it would receive, she could expect to have major parts of the leg repaired each year and the entire leg replaced about every two years.

We had heard many stories about how great the new artificial legs were. I suddenly realized that much of the information had been hearsay. People had told us of "someone" who knew "someone" who had read about "someone" who could do all kinds of wonderful things on a prosthesis. I went home, feeling very let down.

I soon was able to put the disappointment about the prosthesis into the category of "life is like that." I was learning we had to be more realistic about what to expect. I had also learned that the efficiency of artificial legs is related to how much of the person's leg is left after the amputation.

Amputees who still have their knee are able to have a better working prosthesis. If an amputation is above the knee, the artificial leg will work best if the stump is long. People with an amputation at the hip have little or no chance of walking well with a prosthesis. I was sorry that only about one-third of Becki's thigh remained, but I was also grateful she had that much.

Although I trusted God through each disappointment, I also learned that it still hurt me to have Becki hurt. She was uncomplaining about the blisters on her stump as she wore the tight-fitting prosthesis. She didn't fret about walking with a funny gait and never being able to run again. But all this bothered *me,* and I wished I were experiencing all of this instead of my daughter.

Because Becki has a great sense of humor, she felt her artificial leg needed a name. She called her first one "Harold the Hairless Wonder." She said to me, "Just think how much money I'll save on razor blades the rest of my life!" The first Harold was succeeded by Harold II and Harold III. Then came "Hard Harvey" and Harvey, Jr., because the outer surface was hard plastic instead of soft foam as the Harolds had been. The next leg was "Norman," because she looked normal when she wore it. "Polly" is her current leg because it's made of polypropylene and polyethylene.

**God Expands My Horizons**
As I became more aware of the world of the disabled, I could see that God was making me more sensitive to others with losses. Instead of focusing on differences between the disabled and the able-bodied, I realize how similar we are. We have the same emotions and intellect. A person on crutches or in a wheelchair is not necessarily deaf or lacking in mental ability, although we often treat the person that way.

One summer Becki's only foot was stepped on and broken. She had to use a wheelchair. As she said, she was "left without a leg to stand on"! People who didn't know her responded as if she were handicapped in every way. I was with her many times and saw that they avoided looking her in the eye. If they spoke, they talked loudly and slowly as if she couldn't understand otherwise. When she and Craig ordered food in a restaurant, the waitress would talk only to Craig, asking him how Becki wanted her meal, even though Becki had just talked directly to the waitress.

Through her wheelchair experience I also learned that many public places are still inaccessible to the handicapped. Becki told me how embarrassed she was when she went to a pizza place with her friends and had to be jostled over a guy's shoulders and very unceremoniously lugged in because no wheelchair ramp was available.

One Christian conference center, where she was speaking with us, has a restroom stall for wheelchairs, but the restroom is on a hill with only stone stairs for access. While that wide stall meets one of the state codes, I'm sure the restroom never has had a wheelchair inside. Entry to other restrooms is often through heavy doors, or a second large door must be held open while maneuvering a chair through the first door.

I've also become very indignant toward able-bodied people who park "for only a moment" in a handicapped space. They never know how much a disabled person is inconvenienced because of their selfishness. They also never know when they may be caught there by the irate parents of an amputee! Instead of venting our anger, however, we now place a politely worded card resembling a parking ticket on the windshields of offending cars.

## Imperfection Is Universal

I have been reminded that God doesn't make mistakes when I've heard Becki say, "I'm not handicapped; I just don't have a leg. Everyone has some kind of limitation." When we realize we all have defects and admit our individual limitations, we more easily see ourselves as fellow travelers in this world. Most people with handicaps want us to reach out to them as equals and to focus on common interests other than their disabilities.

I've become more attuned to how open disabled people are about their handicaps. Some want to talk about it; others are reluctant. I think it helps to be honest and acknowledge that we notice they have problems. Then we should sensitively explore how much they wish to reveal.

People with disabilities can help the rest of us understand

their world. We need to be educated. We're inexperienced. We're afraid we'll say the wrong thing, so we often say nothing. We need them to let us know where the boundaries are.

Becki is the one who helped me feel comfortable with her amputation. The first time she put on shorts to go out in public, I worried about what people would think. Becki wasn't embarrassed, so I eventually learned not to be. It took some time, however, because I even felt strange when I saw her stump around home.

It has taken me years to be able to say "stump" without fishing around to find some nicer word. *Stump* sounds too harsh and like slang. No one seems to have come up with anything better, not even doctors, and Webster's best term is *vestigial body part.*

## Danger: No Leg Ahead

We have had our laughs over the amputation, such as the time when Becki and I were in a shopping mall. An approaching lady pretended not to see Becki with only one leg showing from beneath her skirt. This had happened often with other people, so I thought this time I'd turn and watch the woman after she passed us. The woman did indeed turn to stare at the back of Becki as she walked on through the mall. I looked just in time to see the lady nearly slam into a support pillar as she gawked at Becki.

When Becki was still learning what Harold the Hairless Wonder could and couldn't do, a friend came to our house to show Becki his new moped (a type of motorscooter). Becki was eager to go for a ride and tried to sit on the seat behind her friend. She was wearing her prosthesis, and the knee couldn't bend without her putting her weight on the foot. Harold was sticking straight out! Deciding that this wasn't a very efficient arrangement, Becki pulled Harold off right there and leaned him against a tree. A lady driving by nearly hit a telephone pole as she stared in amazement.

And there was the time that we had driven for several hours across Kansas before we realized that Harold had been lying on the shelf in the back window. Now we knew why people had been looking at us so strangely as they passed us on the highway.

Perhaps the highlight in Harold's life came when Becki and her friends decided he should have a birthday party. She had received her leg on July 12, 1978, so a year later Harold had a party. Invitations were sent, twenty-five or thirty guests arrived in our backyard, games were played and food was consumed by the ton. Harold received the most imaginative gifts that any birthday honoree has ever had. Socks without mates and one-legged panty hose had been made into creative presents.

## Let's Help

Because of Becki's amputation, I've also become concerned for the families of the disabled. While I was an adjunct professor at Talbot School of Theology, I taught a graduate course that focused on the needs of the handicapped and their families. My students eventually would be in church ministries, and I was convinced that they would be powerful instruments to help families of the disabled.

Our class spent each semester learning about the world of the handicapped through assigned reading, my lectures and special speakers. The most significant awareness came, however, as the students got directly involved with a disabled person and his or her family.

Each year Gloria Hawley, mother of two developmentally disabled adults, had our class in their home to share details of family life and special problems. One year some of the class members became concerned for the Hawleys and took time from their busy school schedules to aid the family in concrete ways. They helped get Laura and Craig ready for school in the morning, took them shopping and entertained them occasionally so Gloria and her husband could have some time away.

Christians need to help relieve the pressures of families of the handicapped. Divorce statistics in families where someone is disabled are even more frightening than those for the nation as a whole. It is estimated that four out of five marriages with a handicapped child break up.[1]

A crisis can either strengthen or tear apart a couple's relationship. A husband and wife may become irritable with each other over details that never upset them before. If one mate is preoccupied with the stress, the other may feel left out. If the other person seems unconcerned about the severity of the problem or won't acknowledge that a problem exists, division can result. The sheer physical exhaustion and inconvenience that a crisis or disability creates is enough to strain any marriage. In addition, many families lack adequate finances, friends or recreational time. The rest of us need to tune in to them and offer help.

## The Best Help

The people who most helped me reaffirm that God doesn't make mistakes were those who let us know they cared and were "with us." They were people who put "feet" on their concern. I usually never accept the vague offer of the person who says, "Let me know if there's ever anything I can do." But when a friend has a specific proposal: "I'm making an extra casserole for dinner tonight. When would be a good time to drop it off?" I will usually take advantage of the offer.

Friends of the disabled and their families can help by being encouraging and nonjudgmental. These people are very brave about matters that would swamp most of us. Often, however, we begin to take their courage for granted. We expect them to be marvelous all the time. We forget that they can get upset about the same ordinary things that upset the rest of us. We stop affirming them for their unusual accomplishments that we've come to expect.

When Becki first learned to snow ski after her amputation, she had already been running on crutches, biking with one leg and doing other sports in ways that caused everyone to marvel. Skiing the new way was extremely hard and exhausting, but her friends expected her to be immediately outstanding. Instead of congratulating her for how well she was doing, they said, "Becki, we thought you'd be on a harder slope by now."

Becki is so very active and energetic that people sometimes forget to give her credit for doing all she does under a tremendous handicap. When she is wearing her prosthesis, she is expending at least sixty per cent more energy to carry out the same task as those of us with two legs. Because she balances so well on one leg, we begin to assume that it's no big deal to clean house or cook and serve a meal on one leg.

Most disabled people, including Becki, don't ask for sympathy or acclamation. It's up to us who are able-bodied to be sensitive to their needs, affirming them and letting them be genuine about themselves, their feelings, disappointments and trials. We should let them "pour it all out" to us when they need to and congratulate them for all they do.

## Despite a Good Answer

As the weeks passed after Becki's surgery, I could see how God had prepared us and provided for our needs long before we ever knew we would have a need. He continually verified to me that he hadn't made a mistake. Today, when I look for what his purposes might be, I see some immediate good results from her amputation, such as her ministry with other disabled people. The truth is, though, sometimes I still think, "God, you could have used her just as much with both legs, and she wouldn't have to put up with all the other problems that she has from having only one leg."

Then I remember God's assurance given through Norma, "Becky, I have the feeling you're going to bounce back from this with real victory and vitality. That's my prayer. I love you."

I don't begin to comprehend God's eternal purposes, but I do comprehend that *he is with me.* No matter what crisis or chronic disability my family or I face, this promise is a theme for my life:

Do not fear, for I have redeemed you;
I have called you by name; you are Mine!
When you pass through the waters, I will be with you;
And through the rivers, they will not overflow you.
When you walk through the fire, you will not be scorched,
Nor will the flame burn you.
For I am the LORD your God." (Is 43:1-3, NASB)

# Part IV

# GOD GIVES INSIGHT

# 11

# A CRISIS
# IS UNFAIR

**D**uring *one of our youth-group meetings, Darrin shared* what God was currently doing in his life. Then he concluded, "Bad things happen to everyone. Statistics show that sooner or later, we'll all be a statistic."

At first, everyone in the group laughed. Yet Darrin knew firsthand the ironic truth of his statement. A few months earlier he had been hit by a car while riding his bike. It wasn't his fault; the driver just didn't see him. She didn't intend to cause him harm, but as her car slammed into his bike, his leg was severely broken. He then faced months of life on crutches and a long rehabilitation after an operation to set his broken bones.

After his leg was healed, the doctors realized his leg had a significant bow to it. If it wasn't corrected, one leg would be shorter than the other. He faced further surgery, but the specialists weren't sure if the operation would correct the leg. If the new procedure failed, Darrin's healthy leg would grow as he matured, but his injured leg wouldn't.

It wasn't fair that this innocent guy had to deal with possible physical limitations for the rest of his life. He hadn't caused the accident. He wasn't doing anything wrong or being negligent. It just happened.

Darrin had the insight to see that, although he didn't deserve what happened to him, God had allowed the problem for his learning and growth. Even though he didn't have answers for why this happened to him, it was rewarding to watch Darrin acknowledge God's purpose in his pain and trial. He learned that suffering is unfair, and I can still hear him telling the youth group, with tongue in cheek, "Statistics show that sooner or later we'll all be a statistic."

**Undeserved Physical Suffering**
The truth is, most crises are unjust. Watch TV news for half an hour or visit a hospital to see the unfairness of suffering.

Consider the elderly. I've worked with several older patients who have been abused by their children. One couple's son had beaten them so badly that they had broken limbs and required a lengthy hospitalization. In another incident, an angered son hit his father over the head with a frying pan so viciously that the man was left permanently brain damaged. These elderly people had not deserved this treatment.

Starving children throughout the world are also innocent victims. Add to this, other natural and unnatural disasters, such as plane crashes, terrorism, tornadoes and earthquakes. Recently a jet airliner was hit by a private plane, and many people were killed. The passengers were innocent people who were not responsible for this tragedy that happened to them and their families. But it did happen. And it was unfair!

Another example is Randy, a young patient of mine who was in a serious auto accident. While riding with his friend who was driving drunk, the car swerved off the road and rolled into a ditch. Randy was comatose for nearly six months. When he regained consciousness, he was told the tragic news that he would never walk again. All four limbs were spastic due to severe brain damage. His speech and memory were permanently garbled.

This was awful enough, yet shortly after his accident, his entire family was killed in a private plane accident. No close relatives were left to care for Randy. Where was justice for this young man?

It's unfair that at sixteen cancer entered my life, causing the amputation of my leg. Did I deserve to have my life altered so drastically? I'd always taken care of my body; why did it get sick?

Even though I've come to grips with my disability, I feel cheated at times. Every step I take must be thought out and planned. The spontaneity of climbing, jumping and running is gone. Yes, I know firsthand, life is not fair.

## Undeserved Emotional Suffering

Of course, emotional pain can be even worse than physical suffering. Think of divorce, alcoholism, broken families, sexual abuse, age or race discrimination, broken dreams and feeling that God is silent. Life can be very unfair.

Melinda's mother has had three marriages and is planning a fourth. Melinda and her brothers and sisters have been sexually abused by two of their mother's husbands, and their mother has physically and emotionally neglected them. This is not fair! Melinda doesn't deserve the suffering she is going through—nor the scars she will carry for her lifetime. Why was she born into an unloving and abusing family?

Another example of life's inequities is my friend Jenny who has had numerous miscarriages. She is young and healthy but unable to carry a child to full-term. Her emotional pain is compounded by the large number of women having abortions. How can some women destroy their babies when Jenny can't even have one she wants so much? Why doesn't God give her the gift of a child?

Emotional pain is felt by families when they must decide how to care for their aging parents. Karen loves her mother and would like to care for her at home. But her elderly mother is confused and disoriented. She needs constant watching to keep her from wandering off. She refuses to wear protective clothing but wets the couch and carpet several times a day. She needs help with dressing, eating and other daily functions. On top of this, she argues incessantly. The stress and strain of caring for her mother would limit the attention Karen should give to her own family, but the guilt for putting her in a nursing home is painful too.

Disappointments are also painful. In college Marcie felt God was leading her into social work. She graduated with honors in only three-and-a-half years and then began job-hunting. After over two years of closed doors, Marcie started to question God's purpose for her. Why had he given her a burden to help others and then apparently abandoned her? Why had he allowed her to spend so much time and money getting ready to help? Where was his guidance now? Did God even care?

## Why Me?

For many of us, the natural response to problems and tragedy is, "Why me?" Somehow we feel singled out. We wonder if perhaps God is punishing us for some sin we have committed. Many people really believe that God is vindictive.

When I had cancer, some people told me, "If you would repent and ask God to forgive you, God would take away your cancer." Others said I must not have followed God's formula for healing, so he handed down the sentence, "Off with her leg!" They made God into a celestial Henry VIII.

People who blame God for pain and difficulties perhaps haven't taken enough time to get to *know* God. They may not enjoy him as a close friend. It's important not merely to know about God, but to know him intimately. It's true, we have all sinned, and we need to come before God daily and admit our sins, but personal sin isn't the reason for all suffering.

Some "loving" people have misused the Scripture with me, quoting Exodus 20:5 about God "punishing the children for the sin of the fathers to the third and fourth generation." If God intended to physically punish the next generation, many more people might be amputees. In fact, if you knew my dad, you would wonder why I haven't been whittled away to nothing by now! (Dad, if you're reading this, I'm just teasing!)

Unfortunately, some insensitive people twist Scripture to find a reason for tragedy. They blame parents for a child's birth defect or accuse a crime victim of a sin that must have caused the crime.

Human reasoning will not answer why pain happens to us. We need to remember that God is an infinite God. His plans and designs are much greater than our understanding. We can drive ourselves crazy by trying to figure out the "why" instead of accepting that it "just is."

## Does God Care?

Suffering doesn't mean that God doesn't love us. Actually, none of us *deserves anything* from God, but by his grace he made provision for us to be saved from eternal judgment. In fact, God loves us regardless of our response to him: "He causes his sun to rise on the evil and the good, and sends rain on the righteous and the unrighteous" (Mt 5:45). His unconditional love is not swayed by our disobedience or unfaithfulness.

God's unconditional love for us, however, does not save us from the normal tragedies that come with living in our world. No one is exempt from the difficulties of our humanity. The successful life is not living without problems but learning to cope with the unfairness that comes to us. Instead of pouring our energy into learning "why," we need rather to ask God to help us live and grow because of it. As Kelly Willard sings, "I'm not asking you to take away my sorrows. But I'm asking for the strength to make it through."[1]

Many times we ask God, "Why, why, why?" If we don't find an answer, we feel God doesn't care. We think he is obligated to keep us from anything hard, unless we see a good reason.

**Knowing Why**
I wonder if knowing why would make our suffering any easier to accept. Would Job's ordeal have been any more comfortable if he had known the reason? Perhaps focusing on why is an excuse. We unconsciously say, "Until I understand the reason behind my pain, I'm not obligated to deal with it." We may then become stalled at the questioning stage and never move on to living life *with* the pain.

Having the why answered isn't what we need. The emotional gut-level why is the real issue. We need the permission to say "Ouch! this hurts!" In reality, the question, "Why is this happening to me?" is more a scream made at a moment of pain than a real question.

I ask why when my stump is blistered and my back aches

from wearing my prosthesis. The truth is, I already know why. I just need to say "help" to my Father. My *why* is one way I admit my weakness.

God is eager to meet us in our emotional *whys*. He is ready to listen and help. And we need him most when our pat answers to life's pain aren't cutting it.

Robert Wise, in his book *When There Is No Miracle,* reminds us, "No matter what is happening to you, God is still the Father of mercy. . . . believing that God's mercy is still surrounding your life will lift your eyes beyond the shadows around you; good is just over the horizon."[2]

Even when we don't know the why in suffering or can't see the end result of our pain, we do know that God's grace, mercy and love are constant. Isaiah 46:3-4 states assuredly: "Listen to me, . . . you whom I have upheld since you were conceived, and have carried since your birth. Even to your old age and gray hairs I am he . . . who will sustain you. I have made you and I will carry you; I will sustain you and I will rescue you."

## An Imperfect Present—A Hope-filled Future

We live in an imperfect world. Because Adam and Eve made the choice to defy God, as we all have, our world has fallen. Human beings haven't been content just to know God and have him provide for us. We want to be like God with his power and control. Wanting our own way is the basis for our rebellion against God's authority.

Things are no longer running the way God originally planned. God intended a perfect world, but he also gave people a choice, and we chose not to follow him. Now we are residents of this fallen world and victims of a scheme that has gone wrong. It's important to remember this when we feel we are being singled out by God.

Heaven offers an incredible hope for me. The promise of the

future gives me strength every day. I know heaven is perfect and all that is wrong will be made right. My imperfect body will finally be new. I'm not sure of the form it will take, but I know I will be whole and without my current physical limitations.

Heaven will also be life without sin. I won't have that nagging regret for the things I do wrong nor will I constantly need to ask God's forgiveness. In addition, heaven is going to last forever. It's exciting to realize that I will have eternity to spend with the Lord. Time limits for talking with my friends or great saints from the past won't exist. Neither will I have to hurry up or manage my time—time won't even be a factor.

Best of all, in heaven I'll be as close as I possibly can be to God. Right now, as I live my earthly life, my relationship to him is "long-distance." Christ communicates to me through the Bible, other Christians and prayer. I communicate back to him through prayer, thoughts and action—but I long to actually see him.

It's like my friendship with my girlfriend Sandy, who now lives in Boston. We haven't seen each other for almost six years. We write letters every week, pray for one another and occasionally splurge on phone calls. We send little gifts to each other. I even talk to other people who know Sandy. But she and I are not able to see each other face-to-face or touch each other.

Even without seeing Sandy, I love her very much and deeply treasure our friendship. The day Sandy and I can hug each other again, though, will cause those letters and phone calls to seem insignificant. Nothing can compare with being together.

In the same way someday I'll embrace Christ. And the best part of it is that he'll never go back to Boston. We won't ever have to say good-bye.

## For Now . . .

For the present, however, I need to remember that suffering happens and it is unfair. Pain does not discriminate. Crises in some form will happen to all of us.

One day after my surgery I rode in a car with some high school friends. Jeff was in the driver's seat. He had just lost his mother because of cancer. In the passenger seat next to him was Kris. Her mother, who had been married and divorced three times, had died and her father had disowned her. Now Kris was living alone, with no support, trying to finish high school. In the back seat next to me was Julie, whose mother had been in and out of mental institutions her whole life. Julie's father was seldom home. He purposely had taken a job that required being away for long periods of time.

Finally I looked down at my stump and thought, "At some time in life, everyone has pain and suffering—whether seen or unseen, large or small." Yes, suffering is unfair, but it can be positive if it makes us stop and think.

# 12

# A CRISIS
# MAKES US STOP

**I**t was the day of New Year's Eve, 1981. The sun was bright and the day was warm, so a friend and I decided to go hiking in the mountains near San Diego. While there, we spotted some great climbing rocks. I hadn't yet tried rock-climbing on one leg and thought it would be a great adventure. My friend had done a little rock climbing and said he would teach me.

We hiked to a ledge from where we could start our climb. My friend showed me some moves and holds. I followed his instructions, and before long I was up about thirty feet. I didn't realize the danger I was in by not having proper safety equipment, ropes or even the right kind of shoe.

Before I knew it, a rock pulled out and I went crashing down the mountainside to the ledge thirty feet below. Fortunately, my friend grabbed me before I fell three hundred feet farther.

It was a terrible fall, but I was glad I landed as well as I did. I knew I hadn't injured my spinal cord because I was able to move all my limbs. However, throbbing pain soon made me realize I had fractured both wrists. My chin also was bleeding from a large gash.

As we rushed back to San Diego, an hour's drive away, I was feeling very disappointed. My injury would ruin many of my plans. I was looking forward to driving to Orange County that night to be at my parents' house for a New Year's Eve party. I also planned to go skiing a couple days later with a handicapped ski club. I was hoping to eventually become an instructor. Although I was glad I hadn't been hurt worse, I still didn't understand why God allowed this to happen now and interrupt everything.

The x-rays showed that I had severely fractured my right wrist. Some of the small bones were so dislocated that I needed immediate surgery. My left wrist was cracked in a few places, but it only needed to be immobilized. The deep gash on my chin was cared for by a plastic surgeon.

I phoned my parents from the emergency room in San Diego and broke the news gently. I explained the accident, describing the smaller injuries first and building to the surgical finale. They immediately wanted me transferred to a hospital near them in Orange County.

### New Hospital

Two and a half hours later I lay in another emergency room, in another hospital. Again I thought of all my ruined plans. It was New Year's Eve; in fact, it was now midnight. Some New Year's Eve! The whole day had been spent lying around being tested, treated and diagnosed. I felt frustrated. So far, 1982 was a drag.

Early the next morning I had surgery to repair my right wrist. The orthopedic surgeon had to use five pins to hold the bones in place. We later learned that the doctor didn't even expect my right wrist to heal. He thought he'd have to perform additional surgery to fuse some of the bones.

During the next few days of recovery, I began to rethink where I was headed. I needed to restructure some of my priorities. The accident took me away from all of my supercharged life, giving me plenty of time to reflect and consider things I didn't want to face. I began to think about my relationship with the guy I was dating.

## New Man

At the same time, recovering from that injury provided an opportunity to strengthen a new relationship that had just started. When I was visiting my parents for Christmas, I had met Craig Sanders. He was working in a sporting goods store where I got a backpack. We had a great talk, and the next day he came to see me at my parents' home.

We talked about his outdoor recreation experiences and some of my future plans in the same profession. We really hit it off! He was a warm, Christian guy, and I was very interested in him. However, I was already involved in the other relationship.

When Craig heard of my accident, he came to visit me in the hospital and called me several times while I was recovering at home. Those casual moments together helped deepen this new friendship and gave me hope for a different kind of dating relationship.

One night while lying in bed, I thought about Craig and all his exciting qualities. He not only had spiritual depth and maturity but also liked to have fun. I thought to myself, "If there are men like that out there, what am I doing with this other guy who continually drags me down spiritually, makes me feel inadequate and keeps suggesting that God has no purpose for my life." Being stopped in my tracks and reflecting on that poor relationship led to a break-up after a few weeks. Craig and I were married a year and a half later.

Of course, I never knew all this the day I fell. My accident seemed only to be a big inconvenience that ruined all my plans. I wouldn't be able to ski at all that season because my arm would be in a cast for six months. As an amputee, I needed two healthy arms to guide the outriggers I used when I skied on one leg.

### "Calamity Jane"

The accident also affected my college work. My note-taking for classes that semester looked like a kindergarten project. Because my right arm was in a cast and my left wrist was bandaged, it was difficult for me to do special projects or to get assignments done on time.

The accident limited many other activities. Riding a bicycle to class with both wrists broken was a real trick! It was also a challenge to use crutches, carry books, wash dishes and clean house. The whole experience seemed like such a big bother. Why had God allowed it to happen? Injuring two of my three limbs seemed *very unnecessary*.

I couldn't put on my prosthesis without the power and leverage of both wrists, so my mobility options were limited to one leg and two crutches. But even the crutches posed a problem. Because both wrists were fractured, I couldn't use my hands to bear my weight on my usual crutches. We had to hunt all over the L.A. area to get special "trough crutches" which carried the weight on my elbows and forearms.

One day at a grocery store shortly after my injury, a man looked at me and said, "Honey, you must have had a terrible accident." What a sight I was! I was on one leg. One arm was in a cast and the other wrapped in an Ace bandage. Both arms were extended from my trough crutches as I carried some groceries. I still had a big white bandage on my face where the plastic surgeon had stitched my chin. I felt like a walking disaster.

## The Backpacking Accident

Six weeks before the rock-climbing accident, I had had another freak accident. I was backpacking on my crutches with friends. After we reached the mountain summit, we were goofing around and I was knocked down. I fell on a log and tore several muscles in my lower back. The spasms from the torn muscles put me in such pain that I was unable to move.

After spending a cold and painful night in the mountains at the 10,000-foot level, I was airlifted the next morning by the Sheriff's Search and Rescue Helicopter. I spent a week in the hospital on heavy medication. Then I spent several days in bed at my parents' home, barely able to move.

The irony of my back accident is that I didn't stop to think about why this had happened. I didn't bother to consider why God had taken me out of my routine. All I did was hurry back into my hectic lifestyle and attempt to catch up on the things I'd missed. It took the second accident six weeks later to get me to be reflective.

Maybe God has to work harder to get the attention of some of us tough, self-reliant types. I'm not saying that God is mean and vindictive or that he likes to see us hurt, but sometimes he allows tragedy and crisis to stop us in our busy routine. He

*161*

wants to give us opportunity to think carefully about life and important decisions.

As I look back, I clearly see that if I had continued my heavy schedule of college classes and numerous extracurricular activities, I might have stayed in that bad dating relationship. I probably would have married the other guy, never stopping to think about whether or not he was God's best for me. I would have charged ahead, not taking the necessary time to discover God's best.

*God wants our crises to stop us!* Any crisis—whether physical, emotional, financial or spiritual—takes us out of our regular routine. It stops us cold. One of our biggest struggles is being overly committed. We have 100 million commitments to 5,000 different people. We rush from one activity to another without enjoying what we're involved in. We even resent the people to whom we've made the commitments. Perhaps the over-committed state of our lives is the major cause of our personal stress.

## Obsessed with Activities

Gordon MacDonald, in his book *Restoring Your Spiritual Passion,* writes of our overcommitted lifestyle in this way:

An associate of mine is fond of comparing situations in which one is overwhelmed by good things to do and learn. [It's like] taking a drink from a fire hydrant. A little bit of water from a gentle fountain can go a long way, he says. But put your mouth in front of a flowing hydrant, and things can get dangerous. What could have brought refreshment can also bring injury.[1]

MacDonald goes on to conclude:

And then there comes the inevitable moment when we become aware . . . that we are going through motions, responding to habits. But the busyness is passionless. We are doing more and enjoying it less.[2]

Often the pattern of my life is to be scheduled up to the gills. I frequently haven't had one minute that I could give to another person or project. I have run through weeks and months not even thinking about priorities or how I was spending my time. I just follow through on commitments and keep everybody happy.

Our society has become obsessed with activities. Somehow, we think if we do more, we'll feel complete and content. Our busyness goes deeper than working for financial gains alone; our accomplishments become the core of *who* we think we are. If we aren't occupied every minute of the day, we think we aren't worth as much. So we frantically fill our days in the hope of finding a lasting sense of purpose.

## Activities Blind Us to God

My hectic, crammed schedule can also cloud my view of God. I can become so wrapped up in tasks that I lose sight of his purpose in my daily life. I confuse "important" with "urgent." Unconsciously I make priority choices based on time constraints. I gradually forget God in my busyness. My personal Bible study is cut short, prayer time is skipped and worship experiences are distracted, because, after all, "God will understand." Sometimes it takes a crisis to help me see what is important in my life.

When my husband accepted a church position in northern California, we packed our worldly possessions for the move. We had to leave them stored in a local storage facility in southern California for a few weeks until we found a place to live.

Once we found a home, we called my dad to arrange for the moving company to move our household goods. The day the professional movers unpacked our storage compartment and loaded the truck, they dropped two boxes, breaking all the dishes in one box and ruining some other items. My dad called that night and warned us to expect some damage and to carefully watch the movers as they unloaded. I was furious that someone could be so irresponsible.

For the first couple of hours after hearing the news, Craig and I ranted and raved about these "professionals" being paid all this money and yet treating our things as if they were trash. They seemed uncaring and callous.

It wasn't long before we both grew silent, realizing how materialistic we had become. We were so concerned about dishes being broken that we totally lost our focus about why we were at our new home. Instead of being thankful that God had provided a new church and ministry for us, we were getting caught up in the hassle of moving and being treated unfairly.

We had a long discussion that night about how natural it is to be conformed to the world's standards. It had happened gradually without our even realizing it. We needed to consciously transform our minds, as Romans 12:1 reminds us.

That little, frustrating "tragedy" made us stop and think about our focus. Perhaps if everything had arrived without a scratch or dent, we never would have stopped to reflect on how important "things" had become. As I look around my house at our possessions, I realize these don't last, neither do they give me real happiness.

God used a few broken dishes to take us out of our routine long enough to help us remember something we knew but had forgotten. It's good for small inconveniences to happen. They help us adjust our priorities. How self-indulgent we might become if things always went our way or life was always perfect.

## Activities Blind Us to Others

Our overcommitted lifestyles also blind us to the needs of people around us. When we are consumed with our own schedules, we don't have energy left to care for others. The real tragedy is that we are so busy we don't even notice our blatant neglect.

I thrive on routine. I think if I can plan a perfect schedule, I will live each day without a flaw. My favorite companion is a "Day at a Glance" calendar. I love to make "to do" lists. I get incredible joy from crossing off accomplished tasks. But no matter how organized my days are and how well I plan each week, interruptions always occur. I can either view these interferences as a nuisance in my routine or as an opportunity to see God in a new way and to listen to him.

The first several months after our move were important in my growth. Things definitely did not go my way. After Craig's graduation from a southern California seminary, we began to look for full-time ministry. In a few weeks we received the call from the northern California church. I quit my full-time recreation therapy position in a well-known hospital and prepared to move. I planned to take a couple of months off to get resettled and job hunt.

As the weeks went by, I began to realize that job opportunities in my field were scarce in this new location. I felt confident that God wanted me to work, so I continued to search, assuming the right job just had not come along. I interviewed for the available jobs, but other applicants with better contacts were accepted. My self-esteem took a beating.

As each unemployed month dragged by, my frustration grew and my self-doubts increased. I couldn't understand why God had called us to a place where I was unable to find employment. Surely God wanted me to work full time—or did he?

Being unemployed was very hard for me. I was accustomed to living life at 150 miles per hour all day long. Many times I'd look back at a couple of months and wonder, "Where did the time go? It still seems like January, and here it is April." I had every five minutes of each day scheduled from 6:00 A.M. until 11:00 P.M. Now I began to feel guilty because I was not continually stressed out. Isn't it God's will for us all to work hard and be under pressure?

## A New People-Focus

It was painful not to have a job. I now had to find my worth in other areas. Instead of throwing a job title at people or telling them how busy I was, I could only present myself. I had to search for a new identity.

Being jobless took away all of the rationalizations I hid behind. I now realized how often I had ignored friends and needy people because I was too busy to help. I had made excuses for not being able to do favors because my time was too committed. Now, without a job, I no longer had a reason to ignore my responsibilities to people.

I found myself caring more for the older lady who lived next door. I noticed people who needed rides or meals. I wrote letters to friends with whom I hadn't communicated for months. So, even in the face of feeling useless and unworthy because I was unemployed, I saw God bring about a deeper closeness to him and a new fulfillment I hadn't felt for a long time.

I began to understand what service and obedience to him could be. I was doing exactly what he called me to do, even though it wasn't what I thought I would be doing. I had thought I needed to be a professional with a title in order to serve God; instead, he was now using my simple acts of caring.

I'm not saying we can't serve God and work full-time. My profession is one of helping people, but days and weeks would go by as I just went through the motions with my patients and without genuinely serving Christ. I think God needed to stop me for a few months to help me re-center my life. I needed to ask myself *why* I was living.

Now that I'm not so overcommitted, I've found that my desire for serving has greatly increased. I no longer feel put out when people need something. I'm joyful that God has given me the means and ability to serve others. I'm content to do exactly what God has given me to do today, realizing that, as I wait on him, he'll take care of all our needs, whether financial or emotional.

## Activities Blind Us to Problems

Often we are tempted to do, do, do—piling up accomplishments so that we feel worthwhile. But maybe we are missing opportunities to learn, to enjoy necessary quiet time, to prepare for the next life stage or to face problems that need correcting. Crises, no matter how big or small, offer these opportunities.

The Martins appeared to be a very spiritual family. Both parents were church leaders in positions of respect and authority. Although they both had full-time careers, they each put in at least fifteen hours a week on church activities. The children were active in church, Sunday school and the youth program. Their family cars were going between home and church many times a week. But it all was a Christian veneer. Underneath the facade were many problems.

Finally their oldest daughter was arrested for cocaine use. It caused a big scandal in the community, and the parents were very embarrassed. The family was forced to stop pretending that life was dandy and to realize they had to deal with several serious problems. Their daughter's arrest was the impetus to get the entire family into much-needed counseling.

Incredibly, instead of receiving criticism from their church friends, they were loved and supported. Other people in the church opened up about problems with their kids. A new freedom was released so they all could struggle together as Christian parents.

There's a paradox here. On the one hand, it's frustrating when negative things happen to us, but it is exciting when God uses them to change us. When a crisis destroys life's comfy routine, instead of automatically grumbling about our disrupted plans, maybe it's time to stop and look expectantly for God's lessons. If a loved one dies, a child is sick or a tire goes flat on the way to work, we may miss some activities, but we can use those potentially frustrating times to ask, "God, why have you stopped me? What is it that you're trying to convey to me?"

## He Makes Me Stop

A familiar psalm impacted me in a new way during my struggles with unemployment:

> The Lord is my shepherd. I shall not be in want.
> He makes me lie down in green pastures,
> he leads me beside quiet waters,
> he restores my soul.
> He guides me in paths of righteousness
> for his name's sake. (Ps 23:1–3)

I was sitting in church when this psalm was read. The words "He makes me lie down in green pastures, he leads me beside quiet waters" hit me with a new force. They made me realize that often God makes me "lie down" for my own good. Naturally, I want to get up and run. I have important things to do.

I really identify with those sheep. I'm sure they thought they knew best. They saw some green grass nearby, and they wanted to run over and eat it. Yet the shepherd said, "You've eaten enough. You need to stop and digest it." The imagery of the shepherd *making* his sheep rest is very strong. God, our Shepherd, is doing that for our own good, whether to teach us or just to restore our souls.

God sometimes takes us away from the busyness of our lives to refocus us on his purpose. God loves us enough to stop us—even when we want to run.

# 13

# A CRISIS
# MAKES US RUN

A few years ago my husband, Craig, taught Outdoor School in the San Bernardino Mountains of southern California. This was a "hands-on" education where the children spent time in the local mountains. Craig taught them how to identify different types of wildlife, trees and other indigenous vegetation.

In one lesson he explained how to tell the difference between a tree squirrel and a ground squirrel. These two types of squirrels look very similar. The easiest way to tell them apart is where their homes are. When a tree squirrel is frightened, he runs up a tree. A ground squirrel, however, runs to his hole in the ground.

In many ways, the same test can be applied to our lives. When crisis or suffering strikes us, where do we run? Where we run tells a lot about what we trust and where our "home" is. Many of us think we would run straight to God when troubles hit. But what do we actually do when we are in a crisis?

## Being a Christian Was Fun

Peter, a man I know, grew into his teen years with essentially no religious beliefs. Although his parents believed in God, they never helped him have a personal relationship with Christ. In his late teen years, however, he began to feel God's pull on his life.

While in the Air Force he met a young woman who was a Christian and began to attend Bible studies with her. In a few months he accepted Christ. His new faith was a source of excitement and joy. His prayers were being answered, and his friends became Christians because of his witness. Peter was fired up to serve God for the rest of his life. His future seemed limitless.

During this exciting time of rapid spiritual growth, Peter went skiing with a friend. He wasn't a very good skier, but he was having fun trying every run on the mountain. They showed off for each other, seeing who could try the most outrageous stunts. Near the end of the day they saw a great jump. They both thought it would make a terrific picture. Peter's friend skied ahead and got ready to shoot the action, while Peter prepared to flaunt his stuff for the camera.

## God Will Take Care of Me

He got up as much speed as he could. As he went over the

jump, he threw his head back. Unfortunately, as an inexperienced skier, he landed on his head rather than his feet. He felt a sharp, stabbing jolt as his body struck the ground. Suddenly everything was numb. He couldn't move his arms or legs. He wasn't in any pain; he just wasn't quite sure what had happened. His first thought was, "I'm O.K. God is going to take care of me. I'm not really hurt that bad. I'll be fine. God will heal whatever is wrong."

The ski patrol got Peter off the mountain and down to the first-aid station. He was then rushed by ambulance to the nearest hospital. Soon he was told the shocking news that he had broken his neck. The doctors didn't have much hope that he would ever walk again.

He lay day after day in the Striker frame, a contraption used at that time in which spinal-cord-injury patients were strapped for the early months of recovery. The patient was suspended between two pieces of stiff canvas and turned alternately to lie face-up for two hours and face-down for two hours. Peter was completely dependent upon caregivers for the months he was in the Striker frame. Eventually he graduated to a regular hospital bed and a wheelchair.

At first Peter was buoyed up by the faith of his Christian friends who came to visit. His friends told him, "God's going to heal you. You'll walk again. Just have faith and wait."

## God Failed

As the weeks grew into months, Peter's faith began to wane. His friends stopped coming to see him. They, too, couldn't understand why God hadn't healed him. Peter began to feel alone and empty. He asked God, "Why have you allowed this to happen to me?"

He finally began to feel as though God had blown it! He had given his life to God—and God had given him a wheelchair.

"What kind of God are you?" Peter fumed. His frustration grew into bitterness as he acknowledged that God apparently wasn't going to heal him. At one point Peter attempted suicide when he realized he would be disabled for the rest of his life.

Instead of trusting God to use his situation, Peter ran from God. He gave up his beliefs and decided to be in control by depending *only* on himself and *never* on God again.

Peter ran from God for more than ten years. He became a successful attorney, owned a beautiful home and boat and traveled around the country demonstrating sports and fitness programs for the disabled. Yet he was empty and unhappy.

Then Peter again began to look to God for meaning in his life. He saw that life means nothing without faith in Christ. Without someone bigger than himself, he had no purpose, no happiness or contentment. Now that Peter is in the process of turning around, he realizes God has been there all the time, waiting for him to stop running away.

### I Can Handle This Myself

If you are like me, you probably run different directions at different times, depending on the type of trouble and trial. In little things I tend to turn to myself. I can handle it when the car runs out of gas, when I forget the coupons for the grocery store or when I oversleep in the morning. But when big traumas hit, I *have* to trust God because there's no way I can handle them on my own.

What an inconsistent squirrel I am! One time I run to myself; the next time I run to God. True faith, however, is when I trust God in every situation, running to him every time.

Fortunately, God loves me in spite of my inconsistency. No matter how many times I run to myself or to other people, he is always waiting for me. It's never too late for me to turn around and find him waiting with open arms.

The amazing thing is that, even if we've run from God for five or ten years, the moment we stop, he's right there with us. We don't have to run back for five or ten years to find him. In spite of the fact that we don't recognize God is there, he is. Although Peter refused to acknowledge God, that didn't mean God left him.

## Yell, If You Must

Even if we're mad at God because we feel he has disappointed us, he wants us to keep talking to him. I really believe God would rather have us communicate with him while we're screaming and angry, than not at all.

Sometimes we assume God can't love us if we don't feel love for him. We reason, "Until I am able to be at peace with this difficult situation, I shouldn't let God know about it." We wrongly think that only after we've wrestled with our problem and accepted it, can we again enjoy fellowship with God.

This faulty thinking diminishes our view of God, making him too small to deal with our anger. It separates us from his support. If we feel we must protect God from our doubts and frustrations, we are then left alone, without his perspective. Unfortunately, we are most vulnerable when we are isolated. Without communication with God, we soon will feel overwhelmed by our circumstances.

Nothing destroys a relationship faster than noncommunication. God wants to bring good to all aspects of our lives, but he's unable to do that if we won't relate to him during the hard times. He won't force himself on us.

Dennis and Michelle are good examples of the importance of communication during difficult times. Regrettably, they did not learn this truth soon enough. Their difficulties started soon after they were married. Dennis was pursuing a graduate degree in education and working evenings as a tutor. Michelle worked full-time as a registered nurse, but her salary was barely enough to pay for the essentials. They both were raised in upper-middle-class families and found their tight budget difficult to live with. Frequently, they had to postpone purchases in order to pay monthly bills.

One day Michelle came home from work to find Dennis setting up a new stereo system. He excitedly explained his bargain and said they could pay for it on credit. "Besides," he rationalized, "we need to start building a credit history if we ever want to purchase anything big."

Michelle was angry that Dennis hadn't talked to her first, especially since she was earning most of the income. But she ignored her strong negative feelings and tried to share the excitement Dennis felt.

A few weeks later Dennis went on another buying spree. This time it was new clothes: two designer suits, plus several ties and dress shirts. He wrote a check which he later had to cover with money from their meager savings account. Michelle was livid with anger at his selfish spending and decided to give him the silent treatment. She sulked off to the bedroom to nurse her wounds. She brooded over how hard she worked at the clinic and around their apartment. She felt she pulled more than her fair share in the marriage.

**Retreat into Separation**

Dennis didn't realize the deep hurt and resentment that was building in Michelle. He assumed she simply was tired and went to bed early. The next day, unaware of the tension his extravagant purchases caused, Dennis bought a pair of expensive shoes to complete his wardrobe. Michelle came home from work and saw the shoe box on the living room floor. Without speaking a word, she walked out the door and drove to her parents, who sympathized with her. She decided to stay with them until her "irresponsible husband" learned his lesson.

Meanwhile, Dennis was bewildered by her behavior. He couldn't understand why she was so upset. Thinking she needed time away, he didn't pursue her. This only compounded Michelle's hurt and confirmed her feelings that Dennis was selfish and uncaring. She decided she had married the wrong person. Her imagination painted a grim picture as their separation continued. Since she wasn't spending time with Dennis, her perspective became more muddled.

The days ran into months, with neither one breaking through the silent wall. Eventually they decided their marriage was a mistake and got a divorce. Neither one protested. Perhaps, if Michelle had communicated her frustration and anger instead of running away, their relationship could have been saved. Their physical distance and silent separation only contributed to the misunderstanding and confusion.

## Which Way to Run?

A strong parallel can be drawn between these two stories and our reluctance to run to God, even when we think he's to blame for our problems. It would have been better if Michelle had screamed her feelings at Dennis and if Peter had kept complaining to God, rather than running away. God *does* love and accept us no matter how we feel about him. But we need to keep running *to* him—not away from him!

Every day we are given opportunities to run to God. When I was in junior high school, this was easy to do. Each day seemed filled with suffering. I had acne. I thought I was too fat. My nose was too big. I didn't have enough friends. My ears stuck out. I had stringy hair. My fingernails were too short. Besides all that, I had a little girl's body that I thought never would grow up. Each moment seemed filled with agony.

It was so hard to face all the struggles alone each morning

as I woke up. My only option was to give them all to God. As I constantly ran to him, I saw his faithfulness in helping me with those daily problems. This process built a strong foundation of faith inside me. God began to take away my concern about the way I looked and helped me become content with how he had made me. He didn't take away all the problems. I still was not slim enough, my nose was the same size, my ears continued to stick out, and my hair persisted in being stringy. But those things didn't seem as important when I looked closely into God's eyes and saw his purpose for me every day.

Because I saw God's faithfulness in little matters, it was easy for me to trust God when bigger things came along. He was my close friend, and I trusted him with my most intimate secrets. It was natural for me to talk to him about all my problems, big and small. When I was diagnosed as having cancer, it was easy for me to run to God and not to myself.

I wish running to God came as naturally for us as running to the tree is for the tree squirrel. But trusting God is something we learn. It's also something we need to practice daily, so we'll be ready when a crisis comes. By looking to our Creator to meet our everyday needs and to help us through hard times, we will realize that he is always with us, even though we are only temporary.

# 14

# A CRISIS REMINDS US WE ARE TEMPORARY

**M**ost fifteen-year-olds aren't faced with death. I know my friends and I thought very little about it. I was young and healthy, and it seemed as if I had my whole life ahead of me. Death wasn't a lunch-hour topic in high school, nor was it an issue we tackled in class. We must have unconsciously figured if we ignored death, it didn't exist.

Death was introduced very personally to me during my confrontation with bone cancer. Losing part of my body made me realize how quickly life can be over. I had already lost seventeen pounds of myself in three hours. How could I be sure the rest of me would last any longer? I never again could assume I'd live until the ripe old age of ninety-five.

Young people aren't the only ones who deny their mortality; many adults assume that life will continue as is. Why not? Death is so cleverly hidden from us. Sure, we see it on TV everyday, but we know it's not real. That stunt actor will get up as soon as the film is shot.

## Death Is Real

In our country we usually don't see our loved ones die. They're often whisked away to some antiseptic institution so we don't have to face the grim dying process. The dead person's body is then beautifully prepared and made to look alive when we view it at the funeral.

Even the words we use for death mask its reality. We say the person has "passed on," or "is not with us anymore," or is "resting in peace." Using these polished phrases makes it easier for us, the living, to ignore our future deaths.

Actually, death is the only certainty we can all count on. But we don't like to face it now; we'll deal with death when we get "older." The problem is, if we don't face it now, we may be disillusioned and angry when we're dying, especially if we've wasted our lives. We need to look at death now, while we still have time to change our reasons for living.

One advantage of crisis and suffering is to be reminded that we're not on earth forever. Many of us grow up with a theological concept of heaven and hell, but how many of us can actually picture ourselves—or our friends and family—in either place? Although we may claim to believe in life after death, that belief often doesn't change the way we live life *before* death.

## Life Must Be Lived Now

When I was fifteen and learned I would have to have a biopsy of the lump in my leg, I came to 2 Corinthians in my daily devotions. One day these verses blazed at me: "Therefore we do not lose heart. Though outwardly we are wasting away, yet inwardly we are being renewed day by day. For our light and momentary troubles are achieving for us an eternal glory that far outweighs them all. So we fix our eyes not on what is seen, but on what is unseen. For what is seen is temporary, but what is unseen is eternal" (2 Cor 4:16-18).

"Those are great verses," I thought. I underlined them and wrote a little note on the margin of my Bible: "God's promise to me." I tucked that section away in my brain under "neat verses."

About a year and a half later I again came across those verses as I read my Bible. Their true meaning now became very important. As I rode my bike over the brick streets in the peaceful neighborhoods of Urbana, Illinois, one quiet Sunday evening, I suddenly realized the tremendous power of those verses! They were meant for me right now—not when I was seventy or eighty years old. I began to smile as I rode my bike.

The truth was, I *did* have troubles. I now was an amputee. People stared at me. I lived with daily pain and constant inconvenience. I thought, "Here I am riding my bike with one leg, yet the 'eternal glory' far outweighs all of this. God's plan transcends the whole situation of my amputation."

## Focusing on the Important

I began to understand that seeing life from an eternal perspective was the key to contentment in all of life. I needed to fix my eyes *today* on what was unseen. Even though I was wasting away outwardly, I was promised an eternal future that would make the present seem almost trivial.

This truth may not seem obvious to everyone, but it was especially clear to me, since a considerable part of my body had just wasted away. I knew that God was renewing me day by day because I was looking beyond my "light and momentary" troubles. I was not concentrating on my amputation; rather, I was anticipating how God might glorify himself through me.

These verses didn't make me think, "Well, *someday* I'm going to be happy and complete." They changed the way I looked at today. The present had a purpose beyond the experiences of the moment.

My perspective was completely changed. I concentrated more on the spiritual side of myself because only that would last. I had graphic evidence every waking moment of my day that the temporary physical part of me would not last. Now everything good or bad had an eternal value. My missing leg vividly helped me realize that my real home was not earth.

## The "Great Body" Illusion

It's no wonder that our bodies and what we are physically seem so important. As we watch TV, read a magazine or look around our world, it doesn't take long to realize how much we focus on our bodies. We are bombarded with the idea that possessing a great body brings success in life.

Tragically, it seems that everyone *else* is beautiful. Having a great body is an illusive goal just out of reach. We look at ourselves and think, "If I'm going to be successful and achieve, I have to get my body in shape. I must exercise, diet and look good—not for my own enjoyment but in order to compete with everyone else. If I don't have a great body, people aren't going to like me and I'll be a failure."

For this reason, plastic surgery has become amazingly popular. TV and magazine advertisements abound, telling us we can be happier if we have our bodies realigned: "Call Dr. Schmo and he'll make your face prettier, your body slimmer, your breasts bigger and your nose smaller." We trade our money for perfect bodies, so that we can fit in, be liked and love our-selves—we hope.

I have a girlfriend who has had breast-enlargement surgery, expecting that this would help her self-confidence. Unfortunately, this painful and costly surgery backfired. Now my friend feels her breasts are too large, and she is extremely self-conscious. Plastic surgery is not a magic cure for a poor self-image.

## Dropping Out Won't Help

Perhaps at one time you were satisfied, or less concerned, about your appearance. Then something happened—an accident disfigured your face, hearing loss requires you to wear aids, osteoporosis has given you a humped back or weight gain has made your clothes fit tightly. You have started to hate yourself because you feel others are put off by your looks or by your assistive devices.

The tragedy of all this body focus is that if you have trouble accepting yourself, you won't reach out to love others. You may find it easier to stay at home than to be with people and serve others. You may become truly disabled emotionally or spiritually because you have limited yourself.

By the time I was in high school, I sometimes became consumed by external things rather than my relationship with God. I relied on my athletic accomplishments, my looks or my popularity. When I didn't get my energy and enthusiasm for life from God, I depended on other people's compliments.

Many times my looks or performance distracted me from depending on God. I didn't need him because I had myself. I was "together" by the world's standards—five feet, eight inches tall; athletic; blond hair; blue eyes; size twenty-seven Levi jeans. I had many friends and I went out with a variety of guys—I was a nice person in the world's eyes.

As adults we sometimes focus on the cars we own, where we live, the social and economic level of our friends or where we vacation. When our life is built on acquisition and competition, someone always has more or is better.

Our former neighbor, who earned a much higher salary than the other men around us, arrogantly said, "I don't try to keep up with the Joneses. I *am* the Joneses!" Straining after success distracts us from God's real purpose for us and interferes with the deep need we have to be close to God.

## No More Dark Glasses

Many things started to change after I lost my leg. Much of my competition with other people decreased at the same time that my compassion for them increased. My self-consciousness about the way I looked and what people thought about me vanished as I realized Christ's powerful presence in me. These other things really didn't matter. It was as if I'd been seeing through dark glasses for all these years, being influenced by the world's standards.

One of my distractions was my clothing. I had worked since I was fourteen and paid for many of my clothes. I always wanted every outfit put together perfectly. I spent time each night planning what to wear the next day. I kept a list of the clothes I wore to make sure that I never wore the same combination within a six-to-eight-week period.

This was such an obsession for me that I felt frustrated if I forgot to write down what I wore. What if I wore it again? People would think, "She's a slob!" I was horrified that somebody might see me in the same outfit too soon. I laugh now, asking myself how I expected other people to remember what I had worn from day to day when I couldn't.

After my amputation the dark glasses were taken away. Suddenly I could see who I really was and how ridiculous my worries were. God began to change me then, and he continues to challenge me in this area. My amputation is a constant reminder that my physical body is temporary and unimportant compared to who God has made me to be.

## Lori's Light

Lori helped give me this new perspective. She lived in the same dorm at Taylor as my sister Brenda. I met Lori after my second biopsy, when I still thought I would not lose my leg.

Brenda had met Lori in drama class when they did modern dance exercises as a team. Brenda was amazed at Lori's determination even before she learned that Lori was doing all those exercises and dance moves only weeks after having had abdominal surgery. My sister thought, "Wow! She's really motivated."

Brenda later discovered that Lori was dealing with more than simply recovering from abdominal surgery—she had terminal cancer. In fact, her unusual type of cancer was affecting most of her family. Her older sister had just died from it, her father was suffering severely from the same cancer, and her younger sister had strong indications of developing it.

During surgery, Lori's doctors had confirmed she had the same kind of inoperable tumors from which her older sister had died. Lori knew the agony and pain she would have to endure. She had just watched her sister go through it.

Upon first meeting Lori, one would not know of her deep emotional and physical pain. She was a talented, intelligent, beautiful girl with gorgeous dark hair and sparkling eyes. She was a vibrant Christian who loved the Lord and desired to serve him in every way. Ever since she was very young, she had been singing and traveling widely with her family's gospel music ministry.

The exciting part about Lori was that she had a ministry

*185*

everywhere—on stage, in class, in her dorm and even in the hospital. She would often share God's love with doctors, nurses and especially other patients. The Lord opened up doors of ministry and she walked through them. Lori was bold and excited about her relationship with Christ and the difference he made in her life.

It was evident that her strength had come from taking her eyes off her own suffering, even though she had every right in the world to feel sorry for herself. She consciously focused on God and other people instead of herself. God blessed her obedience and dramatically used her to touch others. Her faithful trust and unusual life focus was a model for me as I faced the outcome of my bone tumor.

## Terminal at Age Nineteen

After my amputation I often visited my sisters at Taylor and always included time with Lori. Lori and I spent hours together, talking about the things God had taught us. We had so much in common. We stayed up late many nights, discussing our benefits and the new insights we had gained. Neither of us would have traded what we now had for physical health or wholeness. We shared the excitement we both felt for eternity—our real home. God was much bigger than all of life and the things here that could drag us down.

We felt called to a ministry that would have eternal effects. We weren't consumed by what we had to do each day—passing a test, choosing what to wear, having a date for Saturday night. Our "eternal perspective" greatly changed our focus on the present.

We often discussed God's meaning for life and imagined what death would be like. As we talked, I felt sorry for Lori because I knew she was dying. She was only nineteen years old. I kept thinking, "She should have so much ahead of her, but now she will never be married or have children. She won't get to have so many things that life has to offer." Yet she was eager and excited to die—not simply to get rid of her pain and suffering, but to be with Christ. It surprised me when Lori said she felt sorry for me, because I still had a long life ahead with one leg and I would have to deal with that every day.

I was always amazed to see that Lori's relationship with the Lord was so real that everything else was just a dim reflection to her. All the things she wasn't able to do didn't matter, because she knew in a short time she would be living eternally with Jesus Christ. The reality of heaven gave her great joy and excitement.

### Sorry for Whom?

Because Lori knew she was to die soon, she used every single minute as if it were her last. She wanted to make the most of what God had given her.

She told me about one trip to the doctor for a check up. Everywhere on her chart her condition was marked as terminal. She could tell by the way the nurses and doctors treated her that they felt sorry for her.

"She's terminal. Isn't that too bad? It's tragic that this young girl is faced with this terminal illness," their body language and knowing looks communicated.

She told me she felt sorry for *them.* "Because," she observed, "I realize I'm terminal, but they haven't acknowledged they are. We all are terminal the second we're born."

Then she continued, "I'm no closer to death than anyone is. No one knows how long he or she is going to live, yet everyone thinks it must be at least another fifty years. They assume they've got some more time to get their lives together, start serving God and do what is really important."

Then, rather matter of factly, Lori said, "You know, I know

I'm going to die soon, and so I'm using every single day to serve God with the gifts and abilities I have. I feel sorry for other people who don't realize they have a limited amount of time." Lori taught me so much about death—or, I should say, life.

## Harold and Timmy

Besides serious talks, Lori and I also had fun together. I had named my first artificial leg "Harold, the Hairless Wonder." Lori followed suit and named the tumor in her stomach "Timmy, the Tumor." Then she joked that her other little tumors were the "Thessalonians."

It wasn't morbid humor; it was a practical way to deal with our problems. It was easier to make light of our hard situations than to dwell on the painful things.

Lori's tumor in her abdomen grew so big that she began to look pregnant. She even had to wear maternity clothes. People would smile at her as if they were thinking, "Isn't that exciting, you have a new little life within you." They had no idea that it wasn't life, but *death,* that was growing inside her.

Even during this embarrassing physical state, she was able to be humorous. One time she gave me a picture that someone had taken of the two of us. Underneath she had written, "The Lump and The Stump."

As the months went by, Lori's pain increased and so did her medication. She was less active and spent more time in the hospital. I moved away when she was still quite sick. I knew I would never see her again here on earth.

About six months later she did die. Although it was an extremely sad day for me because I loved her, I was also excited for her. I knew she was in heaven with her best friend, whom she'd been longing to meet face to face. She was now smiling painlessly, enjoying a new body and a life much greater than the one she endured on earth. One of the beautiful things about being a Christian is knowing we never really say good-bye to people who love God. We'll get to spend forever together.

## A Reminder

A verse that shapes my daily priorities is: "Do you not know that your body is a temple of the Holy Spirit, who is in you, whom you have received from God? *You are not your own;* you were bought at a price. Therefore honor God with your body" (1 Cor 6:19-20, emphasis mine).

Living with any chronic suffering or long-term problem can be a spiritual string on our finger, reminding us of our heavenly home. Each morning when I put on "Polly" (my latest artificial leg), I am reminded that I'm not going to last forever. When I fatigue easier than other people, I know just how temporary I am. When I get blisters on my stump from my prosthesis, I realize that this body is mortal.

I no longer am tempted to find my happiness and content-ment in what I look like or how well I perform physically. Rather, I try to glorify God in every situation, whether big and exciting or as mundane as doing the laundry. When I'm doing everyday things as a service to God, they actually have an eternal value because I'm doing them to honor him.

## Aging Forces a Change

Older people are easily reminded they are temporary because of the sufferings that come with aging. I once worked with many eighty- and ninety-year-olds who either were coping with chronic illness or in the process of dying.

Amazingly, many elderly people look alike. They all have white hair or none. They wear glasses or have poor vision. They are weak, their skin is wrinkled and their bones are frail. Often you can't tell the ethnic difference—a Gonzales looks the same as an Anderson. I cared for patients who were incredibly rich and patients who were very poor. Either way, they were aged.

Some patients had been very renowned when younger. One man, Dr. Williams, had been a well-known surgeon and had been instrumental in many medical discoveries. Now he had Alzheimer's disease and couldn't even remember his name. He often didn't recognize his wife and confused me with his daughter. He had forgotten his important professional accomplishments.

## Rising above the Ravages of Aging

The one distinction I saw between patients—regardless of their particular illness, race, wealth or fame—was how they handled this final crisis. While all were faced with life being temporary, some were angry and resentful, but others had a hope that transcended their immediate situation. The patients with hope knew Christ personally and had an eternal perspective. They had trusted God their whole lives, so it was natural for them to continue to hope in him as they neared death. Even if they were experiencing tremendous suffering, I could see the peace in their faces.

One dear patient named Ethel endured incredible physical pain. Because of her illness, she had to lie completely flat. Her legs were paralyzed, and she was essentially helpless. Cataracts clouded both of her eyes, so that she was unable to see TV or read. All she could do was lie in bed and talk.

Each time I treated Ethel, she would recall her life: a simple childhood brimming with curiosity about God's creation, her young adult life filled with a growing knowledge of Christ and her mature years of seeing Christ answer her prayers. As she reminisced, she had a deep love for Christ and glowed with hope for the future.

## Anger or Joy

Patients like Ethel were a real joy. Unfortunately, I met many angry patients who were disillusioned with their aging and dying process. Some had lost their money, or it hadn't given them the happiness they expected. Age had stolen their beauty and energy. Face-lifts and tummy tucks couldn't stop the inevitable. Their independence was gone.

Many had lost their friends through death or by driving them away with their hateful, resentful attitudes. They were neglected by uncaring family members who kept busy elsewhere. Some family members and friends avoided the terminal patient because of their own uneasiness with death. It was common for patients to tell me they rarely heard from their children who they said didn't seem to love them anymore. Many felt cheated by children or a spouse for whom they had sacrificed earlier.

Opal never saw her children or grandchildren, even though they lived in the same area as the hospital. They apparently felt uncomfortable visiting her because a stroke had left her unable to speak. Each birthday, Mother's Day and Christmas she received a dozen long-stemmed roses from her family—but no visitors. One day when the flowers arrived, I found Opal sobbing uncontrollably. The roses only reminded her of her loneliness and the rejection by her "loved ones."

## The Big Zero

My patients who died angry were resentful because they had been fooled all those years. They had given their time to fame, money, a big house, a family and a job. But it all amounted to a big nothing.

Marvin was dying from rapidly spreading brain cancer. He was a difficult patient to deal with. He had been an important businessman who had never given much thought to death. Now, suddenly, he was gripped by the inevitable. He com-

*191*

plained constantly about his business partners, his doctors, the nurses, other therapists and even me. Nothing was right. No one could please him. He was an angry man.

Deep down, he was really angry at himself. He had wasted his whole life on things that didn't matter. Now it was almost over. He had no hope for tomorrow. In fact, tomorrow was a big, frightening question mark.

Death is extremely scary—a vast unknown for those who don't know Christ. But for those with an intimate walk with Christ, dying is going home.

## I'm Homesick

As a very young child I had learned that death was just going home. I went with my father to visit Nellie, an elderly woman in our church. I loved Nellie, but I was uneasy about seeing her. I knew she was very ill, and I didn't know what to expect. As soon as I walked into her room, though, I could tell she was at peace. She was quietly radiant, waiting to see Christ. It was obvious to me that she was looking forward to seeing her best friend.

Nellie was in great pain and very helpless. She was thin and boney, and I thought how awful it was to be that way. I held her fragile hand as she said, "One of these days, Jesus is going to call me home, Becki. I can't wait. I hope he doesn't put it off much longer, because I'm homesick."

A few days later, this wonderful saint died. Hers was the first funeral I ever attended. As I saw her body lying there, I wasn't sad. This was what she wanted. She would be with Christ.

I'm thankful I had the experience of Nellie's funeral, because about four years ago my Grandpa Christon died. He was a wonderful man who had a very simple, yet deep, faith in Christ. When I saw him lying in the casket, I was sad because I would miss my grandpa. I loved him dearly; he had enriched my life in many ways. But I also was happy because I knew he was finally all he was supposed to be. His face looked blank because it was no longer filled with his spirit. But I knew his new face in heaven was filled with the radiance of Christ.

## Why Age?

Philip Yancey's book *Where Is God When It Hurts?* helped me deal with my disability and to work more effectively with aging patients. Yancey talks of an older woman who asked a minister why people have to grow old and go through the humiliation of becoming weaker, getting gray hair, losing teeth, getting arthritis and becoming dependent. She wondered why people can't just live a certain number of years and then simply die. Why do they have to suffer with aging?

The minister answered:

"God has planned the strength and beauty of youth to be physical. The strength and beauty of age is spiritual. We gradually lose the strength and beauty that is temporary so we'll be sure to concentrate on the strength and beauty which is forever and so we'll be eager to leave this temporary, deteriorating part of us and be truly homesick for our eternal home."[1]

The wise minister's statement sums up the important reasons why we suffer afflictions. If we didn't, we might be so content to stay the way we are, we'd never look beyond today. God has so much more for us. He doesn't want us to be satisfied with the mere existence we have now. He wants us to be complete and to look forward to being with him.

Crises remind us that we are temporary. Realizing that we are temporary helps us to look at the end of our lives now, while we still have time to change. If we set our minds on heavenly things—not on earthly things—we will live each day with the right motivation (Col 3:2). Acknowledging our impermanence also helps us enjoy and use what we do have.

# 15

# A CRISIS
# HELPS US
# APPRECIATE
# WHAT WE HAVE

**S**hortly *after my amputation, I was riding my bike along* Race Street in Urbana. I looked down at my right leg pumping the bike and thought how fortunate I was that my one leg was so strong and healthy. I watched my muscles moving back and forth. I was impressed with the power and endurance God had given me. I felt thankful to be able to do so much with one leg. I also was grateful that I wasn't lying in bed going through weeks of chemotherapy.

Losing part of my body made me appreciate the three strong

limbs I had left. I had taken my healthy body for granted before. But now, after losing part of it, I realized how fortunate I was that the rest of my body was strong.

My body gives me great pleasure as I realize how wonderful it is that God has given me my physical abilities. I enjoy participating in many sports, such as water and snow skiing, jogging, swimming, roller-skating, volleyball, soccer, backpacking, rock climbing and rappelling. I feel blessed to be able to take part in these activities.

## I Give Pleasure to God

While in college in Indiana, I was out jogging on my one leg and crutches one night and looked up at the deep, dark sky full of stars. "Wow!" I thought, "God is a wonderful Creator." As I ran past the bushes along the roadside, I could hear myself breathing and the crickets singing their evening songs. I realized how similar I was to any other part of creation.

By running, I was doing one of the things God had created me to do. The shining stars and chirping crickets were doing what God had intended them to do. The trees and flowers made visible by an occasional street light caused me to say to myself, "They're content doing what they were created to do. I can please God just by using the physical gifts he has given me. How exciting that even jogging is a form of worship and praise to God!"

At that moment I felt great joy and pleasure in using the abilities God had given me—everything physical, emotional, spiritual and mental that I possessed. My joy wasn't coming from a sense of personal accomplishment but from knowing I was being obedient to God's intentions for me. By using my abilities, I was also giving pleasure to God.

We often have a false sense of guilt related to our bodies. Some of us think our bodies are enemies or strangers which we're not supposed to enjoy. We feel it's prideful to appreciate how we look or what we can do with our bodies.

It's true that many people have fallen into the trap of body worship, which is promoted by the media with inflated promises of perfection if certain products are used. Some become addicted to exercise and dieting to the point of harming themselves; others become bulemic or anorexic from trying to have a perfect body.

We can, however, take genuine joy in what God has given us and use our physical body—whether it meets the world's standard of perfection or not—as a form of worship, just as we would in singing or praying. God accepts the praise of a less-than-perfect body the same as he delights in our "joyful noise" with a mediocre voice or our praying in stumbling phrases.

Our motives become the key to worship. It can be wrong to sing in the choir or teach Sunday school if we are doing it only to be noticed by others. On the other hand, any activity—even making a bed or cutting the lawn—can be holy if done to please God.

When I'm out running, I picture Jesus running with me in his sandals and long robe. I can almost hear his sandal soles slapping the ground alongside me. I turn my thoughts to pray and reflect with him. This is a special worship time for me. I know God must smile, because I'm including him in all I do, not just the activities that seem spiritual or church-related.

**Wonderfully Made**
I'm excited about the body that God has given me. I praise him for the way my body has adjusted to my disability. I realize that much of my new appreciation has come because I've lost part of my body.

A biology class in college strengthened my awe for the human body. My saintly, old professor, Elizabeth Poe, often stopped in the middle of lectures and quoted part of Psalm 139: "We are fearfully and wonderfully made." Some students would giggle, thinking she sounded corny. Yet that verse in the midst of a long intellectual discourse on cell structure or the circulatory system reminded me to praise God for the marvelous way he had made me.

We're wrong if we don't give God credit for the wonderful way he has put us together. We don't need to feel guilty about taking joy in our body as long as we give the credit to God and not to ourselves.

## Technology's Poor Imitation

Our bodies really are a gift. Man's technology is primitive when compared to anything God has created. I know that firsthand from wearing an artificial leg over the last eleven years. TV programs which portray a Bionic Woman or a Six Million Dollar Man as better than God's creation are just stories. No limbs are like those TV limbs.

I was very disappointed when I got my first artificial leg. It didn't even come close to doing what my own leg had done. I'd been pumped up by people's false encouragement about all the wonderful things prosthetics were able to do. I thought I would be fitted with something almost superhuman.

When I tried on that first artificial leg—with the latest technology—it was heavy, bulky and ugly. It didn't have the characteristics of a real leg. No muscles rippled as it moved. It was lifeless to touch. The only warmth it had was from the room temperature. My fake leg was a sorry comparison to my right leg that stood next to it.

Yes, artificial limbs are improving, but they're nothing compared to the way God had "fearfully and wonderfully" made me from the beginning. Each movement with my artificial leg takes extra thought. Its motions are mechanical and predictable.

Spontaneity is not possible, because each step must be planned.

## God's Gift of Adaptation

By comparison, our bodies are amazingly adaptable. I remember how quickly I regained my balance after my amputation. My strength increased in my right leg. My arms made up for the extra weight they now had to carry. The first few times I was on crutches, I continually perspired because of the amount of energy being expended. Within a matter of weeks, however, my body adapted. My endurance increased to meet the new demands, so that now I can easily run two to three miles on crutches.

Even when someone's brain is partially damaged, the human body can compensate. Many times I've watched brain-injured patients make remarkable gains as other areas of their brains have been trained to take over for some of the loss.

Olive was one of my stroke patients who had lost the use of the right side of her body. She felt afraid and depressed because she assumed she'd be dependent on others for all her care. After all, she was right handed; how could she cook and dress herself? Would she ever enjoy needlepoint stitchery again?

Through therapy and rehabilitative training Olive learned to utilize the left side of her body to compensate for her losses. She soon learned to operate adaptive equipment for her self-care and leisure pursuits. Olive was encouraged when her seventy-three-year-old body adjusted so well. Now, although she uses a walker and her left-handed writing is a little less refined, she still lives alone and is essentially independent.

I know wheelchair athletes who have trained their upper bodies to take over for the loss of their lower extremities. They go up and down stairs in their wheelchairs; enjoy basketball, tennis and "running" marathons in adapted wheelchairs; and even ski on mono-skis or sit-skis—all without the use of their lower extremities.

## Losses Make Us Grateful

Our bodies *are* marvelous gifts. Suffering and loss in any area of our life should help us be more thankful for what we still have.

Unfortunately, it sometimes takes a loss for us to realize all that we've been given by God. Losing a leg made me value the rest of my body. Being out of a job helped me thank God for work. Losing my grandfather caused me to appreciate my living family much more. Since we've moved from my family, I pray more for them now than I did before. I want to show them through notes, phone calls and prayers that I love them. I admit it took distance and death to increase the value of my special family to me.

I often don't face my ungrateful attitude until it's too late and the opportunity, special person or blessing is gone. After the fact, I regret my thoughtlessness in not enjoying the moment. Sometimes I am distracted by future goals and activities so that I miss the unique gifts of today.

## The Loss of Not Having

Often we grieve the loss of things we've never had. We desire a gift God has chosen not to give us. Perhaps it's financial security, a child, a stronger marriage or, in my case, a decent singing voice. Even though we've never actually "lost" these, focusing on not having them can destroy us or can cause us to grow in wrong directions.

Financial limitation may not be a concern for everyone, but it was a major difficulty for Robert and Meg. Robert was transferred to the East Coast, where the cost of living was considerably higher than their previous area. Robert's new salary, although higher, didn't allow them to purchase a house. At first Meg and Robert felt resentful. Why had God moved them and then not given them enough money to live by the community's standards? Meg saw other wives driving Mercedes and enjoying local health club memberships while she drove a Mazda and did sit-ups in her apartment.

After a few months, Robert and Meg began to get a new perspective. They saw their financially comfortable friends and co-workers for what they *really* were—usually unhappy. Neighbors worked so hard at earning money that their intimate relationships were a disaster. They had neither the time nor the energy to develop quality relationships. Many had stopped attending church because they were too exhausted from working overtime to get out of bed on Sunday morning.

Meg and Robert found themselves thanking God for what they *didn't have*—money. They weren't distracted by the pursuit of wealth. They enjoyed a deeply committed marriage and family life with their two young sons. In many ways they were much richer than the people they once envied.

## God Meets All Our Needs

Scripture has helped me appreciate what I have and not to fret over what I don't have. The Bible says, "My God will meet all your needs according to his glorious riches in Christ Jesus" (Phil 4:19). It's comforting for me to realize that Christ will meet *all* my needs. He has done so all the years I've trusted him. He may not provide for all my wants but he certainly does provide for my needs. I've found it helpful to think, "If I don't have it, maybe God knows I really don't need it right now."

Of course, that idea can be taken to extremes and cause us to become very lazy and complacent. For example, I might say, "I don't have a job, so I won't look for one!" More often, though,

I fret about whether we're going to have enough money to buy a house someday, pay off the car, meet medical bills, feed and clothe our baby and on and on and on. I need to remember that when we serve God and seek to please him, he is going to take care of our needs. If he doesn't provide what we think we need, he's going to give us the courage and ability to live without it.

When I go running without my artificial leg, people stare at me. Drivers slam on their car brakes and turn their heads. If I don't wear my leg while shopping, little kids mumble to their mothers about that poor woman with one leg. I am not embarrassed or ashamed. I am doing exactly what he made me to do—using the body I have left.

## The Power of Praise

Deciding to be content with what God provides is not natural. When it comes to material things, I tend to want more and better. I have to practice the attitude of being thankful for what I have and consciously work at not complaining about what I don't have.

I know the Bible says, "Be joyful always; pray continually; give thanks in all circumstances, for this is God's will for you in Christ Jesus" (1 Thess 5:16-18). This simple, concise passage is very powerful—when I actually do what it says.

The day I found this verse, I was excited. Here was a very clear guide to God's will. His will isn't what I *do,* but who I *am.* It's a lifestyle, not a job description. A person in God's will is thankful, joyful and prayerful, regardless of the tasks God might give.

Yes, I know from personal experience that it is difficult to appreciate God, be joyful, pray continually and give thanks in all circumstances. It's so easy to become distracted by daily stresses and conflicts. It's not hard to find reasons to complain—or to join in when someone else is complaining.

Complaining is contagious. Have you noticed how easy it is to jump on the crabbing bandwagon when one person starts to complain about his or her bad day? We almost automatically chime in about the things that have also gone wrong in our day.

Even after a church service of worship and praise, I've caught myself moaning about my bad week, how tired I am or how many things I have to do that afternoon. Instead of admonishing me, my Christian friends join in and say something like, "Yeah, last night was horrible, our dishwasher blew up and the kids didn't go to bed until midnight." We go on and on, caught in the trap of griping. Friendships shouldn't be used as an arena for constant grumbling.

## Comparison Trap

Complaining also comes easily when we compare our situation to other people's. Most often we compare up—to those who seem to have a better life: a new car, a nicer house with a pool, the right number of healthy, well-behaved children or a better job. We notice other people's nice clothes or someone else's husband who seems so kind and sensitive. It's not surprising then that we have a "pity party."

Recently when I was at our mall, I noticed the new styles in the stores and began to feel that all my clothes were horribly inadequate. Yet, I couldn't afford any new ones. I went home very depressed because the clothes in my closet were so outdated. If I had never made the comparison, I probably would be thankful for what I have.

When we compare ourselves with people who seem to be less fortunate, we get a better perspective. Then we begin to say, "I'm so rich compared to many people in the world."

When I'm taking care of people who are sick, dying or have disabilities far greater than mine, I have no room for self-pity.

If my patient has both legs missing, who am I to complain about having only one? Or how can I feel sorry for myself when my patient is paralyzed from the neck down? I'm only missing a limb.

If we must compare ourselves, which God doesn't approve anyway, let's at least compare ourselves to people who are less fortunate than we are. God has done so much for us, and he promises to give us everything we need.

## Does God Have a Pension Plan?

Sometimes we are victims of a consumer attitude toward God. We give him our life, but we want to make sure we get something in return. We often think in terms of "employee benefits," or what I call "servant benefits." We ask, "So what are the perks?" We treat our relationship with God like a business arrangement. We don't want him to cheat us out of what he owes us.

What a distorted attitude! What we deserve from God is judgment, punishment and separation. What he gives us is grace, forgiveness and the opportunity to know him. This alone deserves our complete obedience and service. We need to break free from acting like spoiled children, always demanding more.

Obviously, the hardest time to thank God is when we are in a difficult situation. It isn't easy to be joyful if your husband has just left, you have lost a job, you have had a terrible accident or your child has committed suicide. How are we supposed to be full of joy when things are really rough?

## One Negative Destroys All Positives

When I'm in a difficult time, I don't feel joyful about the actual circumstance, but I can be joyful for who God is and remind myself of all I do have. I am happy that God is with me and that he is ultimately in control of the situation. I realize he is allowing the situation to happen. Even though I may never understand why, I get a sense of peace in knowing he loves me and is in charge.

During my pregnancy I was nauseated for weeks. It was hard to feel joyful while I was vomiting! It was easier to feel sorry for myself. I was much less productive than usual and often was unable to make a nice dinner for my husband since the smell of food made me sicker. I was also tempted to mope around because I couldn't go skiing. Instead God called me to be joyful.

I found *much* to be joyful about: I was able to be pregnant, I was married and had a strong relationship with a wonderful husband, and God was with me and our baby as she was being formed. I was thankful for all the needs that God had met in my life. And yet, I was often tempted to throw a hundred good things out the window and concentrate on the one negative— vomiting!

I had to pray for a new attitude, focusing on all the positives. It helped to enlist my family and friends in the process. I had a girlfriend who was also struggling with feeling negative, so we decided to hold each other accountable. When one of us started to complain or focus on the negative, the other would change the discussion to concentrate on the positive.

## The Key to Contentment

Another friend of mine discovered the value of thankfulness and contentment after years of loneliness and depression. Suzanne, in her early thirties, had been frustrated for years by her less-than-adequate social life. Now as she approached her thirty-third birthday, she found singleness unbearable. She desperately wanted to be married and raise children. She often resented her friends' family life and found it difficult to be with her friends when their children or husbands were around. Although Suzanne loved God, she didn't understand why he would allow her to be single. She had so much to offer to a husband.

One night when Suzanne was home depressed, she began to cry and pray. Almost as if a light came on, she realized how self-centered she'd become. Her mind was suddenly filled with the faces of her closest friends. God had given her a wealth of deep relationships to encourage her and help her enjoy life. All of these years she had prayed that God would bring someone "special" into her life—but he already had.

Suzanne changed her focus from desiring a husband to an excitement for the people God had given her. The process was gradual but definitely positive. Suzanne still doesn't have a husband and doesn't know why. But she is no longer depressed and resentful. Through her pain she's learned the key to contentment: appreciating what she has. Her newfound contentment has allowed her to use the byproduct of her pain, which is the ability to comfort others in their pain.

# 16

# A CRISIS
# GIVES US THE
# ABILITY TO
# COMFORT OTHERS

**K**athy had contracted a severe case of polio when she was a child and was paralyzed from the neck down. She, her parents and seven younger brothers and sisters moved into the house behind us when I was four years old. Kathy was about twenty years old at the time and lived in a special room in the walk-in basement of their house.

Kathy could sit in a wheelchair and, with the aid of several apparatuses, move her arms. She also had a special bed that rocked back and forth to help her breathe at night. She was so thin and frail, I could see why her mom had to prop her with several pillows when she put her in the wheelchair. Her mom also had to totally care for Kathy's personal hygiene: bathing, dressing, applying make-up and caring for her hair. Someone also had to help her eat and drink.

She did her schooling by correspondence and by a telephone connection in the classrooms. She graduated from high school and eventually completed a college degree. I admired what she was able to do in her limited condition, but there was so much she couldn't do. She was horribly confined to that one room.

Her younger brothers and I often ran in and out of their house as we played together. I would see her sitting alone in her room and want to visit her, but we would rush on with our games. I thought about taking flowers to her, letting her know I cared that she was unable to get out of the house. But I seldom did. She was friendly and had a beautiful smile, but I didn't have the courage to carry out my thoughts very often. Besides, I felt what little bit I could do would be insignificant compared to her terrible condition. So I often ignored her.

## "Pass It On"

How differently I'd respond if I could see Kathy today. I would be excited to talk with her about her experiences and struggles. My own life-changing disability has helped me to become a better comforter. As an active, carefree child I didn't comfort Kathy because I hadn't yet needed much comfort myself.

In 2 Corinthians 1:3-4, God tells us that his tenderness for us when we suffer should be passed on to others: "The God of all comfort . . . comforts us in all our troubles, so that we can comfort those in any trouble with the comfort we ourselves have received from God."

I've learned that God uses my difficult situations and hard times to help other people. I'm able to show them the comfort

I've received from God and share the empathy and understanding I've gained through my hard experiences. My struggles don't have to be an end in themselves but are a means to a greater end. This encourages me to look for a purpose in everything I experience.

## Suffering Brings Understanding

Since my amputation, I find myself welcoming people who are handicapped. I'm intrigued by their adjustment and desire to live life to its fullest. Instead of ignoring the disabled, I seek them out and encourage them to continue their fight. My experiences of suffering and daily coping are links to them in their circumstances.

Jesus Christ also experienced trials and suffering and, therefore, can "sympathize with our weaknesses" (Heb 4:15). He knows what it is to be a human and to face testing, so he understands us.

Although Jesus experienced human life and its stress, he didn't go through every *specific* trial we may encounter. For example, he never gave birth to a baby, raised children, married, divorced, grew old or buried his mother. Even though Christ did not face some specific experiences, he did go through the gamut of human emotions related to pain and loss.

In addition, God in his wonderful plan meets our need for support and empathy in our particular situations through other Christians who *have* experienced those things. God's family has many members who have lived through a vast array of life's hardships that Christ may not have experienced.

This concept excites me. Christ isn't simply a model person who lived two thousand years ago; he is alive and living in each of us who seeks to honor God with our lives. Because Christ lives in us, we can bring Christ's comfort to others, as we support them in their pain.

Sometimes hurting people are best helped through a support group where each person has the same struggle. In such a group each person humbly admits he or she is not an expert with all the answers and perfect advice. They are a group of fellow sufferers. In Alcoholics Anonymous, for example, each person shares about his or her own fight to stay sober. All of them admit they have a drinking problem. This personal vulnerability allows others to admit their problem.

What a satisfying arrangement it is that God equips us to help others by means of our own pain and suffering. He first meets our needs, helping us to accept and deal with our crisis as well as giving us hope beyond our circumstances. We then have the privilege of reaching out to others.

## Comforting through Sharing Yourself

Comforting other people doesn't mean simply sending a sympathy card, patting someone on the back or promising to pray. Effective comforting demands personal risk. It means sharing about my own burdens, struggles and failures, maybe even before I've gotten them all straightened out.

Earlier this year as I taught an adult education class at my church, I talked about 2 Corinthians 4:16-18:

> Therefore we do not lose heart. Though outwardly we are wasting away, yet inwardly we are being renewed day by day. For our light and momentary troubles are achieving for us an eternal glory that far outweighs them all. So we fix our eyes not on what is seen, but on what is unseen.

I gave my testimony and shared about the dramatic way God had used this verse to alter my thinking when I faced cancer and the amputation. Then I divided the class into groups of two and encouraged them to share a recent personal experience in which they had to take their eyes off the problem and consciously turn their eyes to Jesus.

As I looked around the room, I saw people chatting, praying and crying. Through sobs Sharon told her partner of her daughter's rebellion and immoral involvement. Her friend listened intently, eyes filled with compassion. She didn't offer advice or biblical directions, but held Sharon's hand as her grief and embarrassment over her daughter's lifestyle gushed out.

Other people in the class shared their struggles and experienced the true comfort and love of Christ. After the class several people thanked me for giving them a forum for their pain. Rarely had they risked like this before.

Although this is a powerful form of fellowship, it is often hard to be vulnerable and honest. The exciting result of sharing our personal struggles, however, is that it frees others to do the same.

It's natural to want to present ourselves as "all together." We find it easy to boast about answered prayers, God's guidance or how we no longer struggle with certain temptations. When we hold these successes up to one another as badges, though, we drive people away and limit their potential for growth.

Unfortunately, some churches and the Christian media are guilty of pushing success instead of showing real humanity. We preach stories of triumph. Many of the listeners hopelessly think they could never be like that. "Success-only" stories cause them to give up rather than keep trying. Sharing struggles and weaknesses binds people together, because they don't have to be perfect in order to relate to each other.

## Suffering Helps You Share Yourself

Even group prayer times can often be superficial instead of promoting openness. In numerous Bible studies I've attended, it's very easy for members to request prayer for other people's struggles: "Pray for my sick grandmother." "Pray for my dad; he's an alcoholic." "Pray for my friend who's failing algebra."

"Pray for Mrs. Smith who is having surgery tomorrow." Asking for prayer for other people's problems is less threatening than asking for our own needs.

A few months ago I was in a Bible study where this kind of comfortable sharing was going on. Everybody was talking about somebody else's problem and not asking for prayer about their own. I noticed Phyllis had tears in her eyes as she wrote down all the prayer requests. Something was really troubling her. Finally, someone encouraged her to share about her need. She said, "No, no, it's not important enough." Yet her tears said it was very important to her.

She finally started talking about the troubled relationship she was experiencing with her daughter. Phyllis couldn't really put her finger on the reason, but she was not able to communicate with her daughter anymore. As soon as she shared this personal struggle, warmth and love began to flow in the group. People supported her, not with advice but by letting her know they cared.

Soon another woman told about her difficult relationship with her husband. A real group with support and compassion then started to form. But first it took one person's tears and courage to risk.

## Sharing Yourself Promotes Growth

Sometimes as I admit my struggle to another person, I'm finally able to admit I need God. Until I verbalize it to someone else, I keep trying to hold it all together, pretending I can handle life by myself. As long as I don't admit my need for God, he is left out of my problem. When I share, it's an opportunity for God to work in me and the other person. Sharing with other people not only invites God into my struggles, but also helps them invite him into their problems.

I may not even know that I've been a help to another person.

Occasionally, after two or three years' silence, I have received a letter or phone call from somebody, explaining that I had been used in his or her life.

After I became a student at Taylor, one of my dorm mates said, "You probably never realized this, but when you used to visit your sisters here, your unembarrassed attitude about your body really helped me accept myself. You see, I'm sort of heavy, and I've always been embarrassed about the way my legs look. I would never wear shorts or go out in a bathing suit because I thought I was ugly and fat. But when I saw you going around in shorts or a bathing suit, not afraid of your stump showing, it made me realize how ridiculous I was about my imperfect body. Since then, I've been able to accept many things about myself and realize they are part of what makes me unique."

I never knew I was being that example. But God is always ahead of us as he uses other people to change our lives and vice versa.

### Experiencing Pain Together Deepens the Comforting

Over the past years God has given me a deep compassion for people in pain. I've enjoyed working in hospitals because I understand what it's like being a patient. I'm not just another expert therapist, nurse or doctor giving advice, prescriptions and therapy plans. I may do that, but underneath I understand how it feels to be helpless. I know what it is to lose my independence. I've experienced tremendous physical pain, and I know it's not going to go away. God has given me opportunities to turn my pain and suffering into avenues for helping other people.

Recently my father-in-law, Gene, had open heart surgery. He had undergone a similar procedure thirteen years before, and this time the increased risks and critical nature of the operation were a very deep concern to our family and friends. We held vigil in the intensive care waiting room while he was in surgery and during the days that followed. Because of his unexpected lung complications, that waiting room became our second home for eight and a half long weeks. He was near death many times.

During that time I witnessed an interesting phenomenon. Our family and the loved ones of other critical patients became an impromptu support group. Each day we'd gather in that little room to wait for the short half-hour visiting periods to see our patient. As each person arrived, others already there would ask how that one's mother, husband or wife was doing. Then everyone offered encouragement, support or excitement over the status of that particular patient.

Sometimes we all prayed and cried together. Strangers became temporary family, bound together by fear and concern. Each of us became vital to the mental and emotional well-being of the others. After all, who was more qualified to share their sadness than others in the same situation?

In many ways that fourth floor ICU-CCU waiting room was the meeting place of a micro-church body. It gave us the opportunity to help and be helped during a time when we all felt very out of control.

## Comforting beyond Your Experiences

God may use us in other people's lives in ways that are different from our own personal suffering. Any difficulty in our lives broadens our ability to care for other people. Even smaller hurts and disappointments can become meaningful tools to reach into someone else's life. For example, I had cancer and an amputation, so naturally I understand cancer patients and other amputees. But I also understand people who experience other kinds of loss.

Recently my friend Connie started to tell me about her divorce. Although I've never gone through a divorce, my heart began to swell with tears. I felt her loss, grief and despair. This doesn't mean I "know how she feels," but I've had some of those same emotions. My experiences of loss help me to feel her loss. When I pray for Connie, I ask God to comfort her and help her feel loved during this lonely time.

## Comforting from Your Experience

I remember my feeling of failure when I didn't finish college in the four years I figured it should take. *I* had my life all mapped out on a certain timeline. Because I attended three different schools, however, I took four and a half years to graduate and that felt like failure to me. Taking a little longer to graduate may not seem like a disaster to some people, but to a highly structured person like me, it was a real setback.

This feeling of failure, however, has helped me to understand kids in our youth group who don't meet the high standards they set for themselves. I can empathize with my friends who have professional failures. If I had never felt failure, I would only be able to give pat advice about how to succeed. But because of my own experiences, I can love these kids and my friends, feel their failures and reassure them that God is in control.

Even my period of unemployment has had a positive side. God has given me a genuine understanding and compassion for other people who are no longer in the work force—homemakers, retired people, people between jobs. I can encourage them to see that God's identity for them is much greater than a job. Who we are in Christ transcends our title or salary. I can care for them because God has met my needs and given me a feeling of significance far greater than any job I ever had.

## Misconceptions Stifle Comfort

Sometimes Christians have the misconception that we

shouldn't struggle or feel emotions deeply. We often believe that depression, anger and grief are sin. Trusting God, however, does not mean denying our emotions.

Without acknowledging our real experiences and feelings, we might miss out on God's help. We could end up relying on ourselves and our own abilities. We might say, "I can handle it. I'll just keep smiling. Everything's going to be O.K."

We need the honesty to cry out, "Hey, God, this situation stinks. I don't like it!" If we keep God at arm's length from our real problems, he can't give us the support we need. When we stop hiding behind our own attempts to hold it all together and admit, "I don't like it! This makes me mad! It depresses me!" he is able to help us.

A picture hanging in our living room illustrates this idea. It's a watercolor of fifteen ducks walking along in front of a house. Some of the ducks are lined up very neatly and walking in a row, all following one after another. The ducks in another part of the picture are all bunched up and looking confused. The scene reminds me of my life. Parts of it may be under control, but other parts are all jammed together and disorganized. Those are the areas in which I need to say, "This piece of my life is all confused, and I can't get it straight. I need you, God."

**Suffering Allows People to Serve**
Admitting we have needs is part of being the body of Christ. All of us have weaknesses as well as abilities. We need to cooperate, complement each other and let others know they are needed. If we function independently, other people get a signal that we don't need them. They aren't important.

During my pregnancy, Craig's parents came for a visit. I was nauseated much of the weekend. Anne, my sweet mother-in-law, did my washing and ironing, cooked, mopped the floor, made my bed and in general kept up the place. That was hard for me because I like to be the "perfect hostess." I want to keep my house clean myself and prepare wonderful meals. I don't like my guests working around my house. Yet, for Anne, that was the greatest thing she could do. Helping me made her feel she was needed and part of the family.

Many times I've been guilty of shutting people out and making them feel I don't need them because I've got it all under control. I've got all my ducks in line. The problem is, sometimes I do that with God as well.

When I don't admit I need God's help, I keep him out. But he patiently waits to be invited to share in my life. When I do let him in, he can give me what I need so I can honor and glorify him as I share his comfort with other people.

**Sharing the Hope**

A few months after my amputation a nurse from our church called me about Calvin, a sixteen-year-old patient of hers. He had just had a leg amputated because of cancer and was so depressed he wouldn't talk. My nurse friend asked if I would visit him in the hospital.

I looked forward to meeting Calvin and sharing what I knew about life as an amputee. In that part of Illinois, there weren't many young amputees. Before my surgery, I couldn't locate any others my age to learn from.

I hadn't yet been fitted with a prosthesis, so I went to the hospital on crutches. It was a warm day and I wore shorts. Of course, my stump was showing.

I walked into Calvin's room and introduced myself. He barely looked up but did raise his eyes a little and saw that I was on one leg. That caught his attention enough so he listened to what I said next.

"It looks like you and I have something in common," I ventured. "I see by the lump under your sheets that it's even the same leg."

He seemed horrified that I mentioned the lump, but I went on, "I used to call mine a basketball. But don't worry, the swelling eventually goes down. I'm waiting now for my stump to heal enough to get fitted with a fake leg."

Calvin shifted uncomfortably and didn't look at me, but he seemed to want to hear more. I kept talking about my experiences as an amputee. At one point I referred to the amount of stump I had left and what that meant for the fitting of an efficient prosthesis.

"How long is your stump?" I asked. He didn't answer, so I said, "Let me see it."

He was absolutely shocked and said, "I haven't even looked at it. And I don't intend to!"

Eventually he shared that not only had he avoided looking at his stump, but he also hadn't discussed the loss of his leg with anyone. He was from another city, so his only visitors were his parents. They didn't talk with him about his amputation either.

I also discovered that Calvin had decided to drop out of life. Although he was a good student, he didn't plan to return to school. When I told him he would still be able to drive a car because he had his right leg, he said his family's cars all had manual transmissions—"You need *two* legs to drive them." He didn't care anyway; there was no place to go and no one he wanted to see.

I could tell this guy badly needed a new perspective, so during my next visits I prayerfully worked at helping him. He needed to grieve over the loss of his leg. He also had to accept the reality that life would be different but he would still be able to do many things.

During my visits Calvin began to feel free to talk about his situation. His depression lifted. He could look at his stump and acknowledge that his left leg was actually gone. He began to think of things he wanted to try to do. He talked about getting his dad to buy a car with an automatic transmission. He decided to go back to school as soon as he was able.

One day as I left his room, his parents were coming down the hall. They grabbed me and couldn't thank me enough for how I had helped Calvin to find hope.

"I'm glad I could," I said, "but I've just passed on the encouragement that God and other people have given me."

It's true, our troubles and crises allow others an opportunity to comfort us. In turn, experiencing pain gives us the ability to comfort others and help them trust "the God of all comfort, who comforts us in all our troubles, so that we can comfort those in any trouble with the comfort we ourselves have received from God" (2 Cor 1:3-4).

# An Afterword

## A MOTHER'S PERSPECTIVE

# BECKI NOW

*Becki brought the house down! The women rose to give* her a standing ovation, and I was again overwhelmed at God's marvelous and mysterious ways.

Becki and I had just spoken together at a woman's conference at Mt. Hermon, a picturesque Christian retreat center in the California mountains. I had spoken to the women at the sessions prior to the final meeting when Becki joined me. After I said a few introductory words, Becki took the rest of the hour to share—with a mixture of humor and honesty—about what God had taught her through her amputation.

I was filled with renewed awe over God's gracious plans. Here was my amputee daughter, now a wife, mother, recreation therapist and youth worker, allowing God to take a potentially tragic experience and turn it into help for others.

Becki is the mother of our healthy, charming granddaughter Hayden, who was also present as we spoke. When the audience broke into applause, Hayden, who was ten months old at the time, started clapping too.

After we finished talking with a number of women following the meeting, Becki drove us back down the mountain to the country-style home that she and her pastor-husband, Craig, have tastefully and inexpensively decorated. In a few hours she would be helping Craig with the Sunday-evening meeting of their senior-high youth group. Later in the week she would spend half a day directing a city recreation program for the disabled.

A normal week for her also includes a few friendly lunches with teen-age girls, helping another teen pick out a birthday present for her dad and listening to a troubled mom pour out her heart about a rebellious son. She writes some letters of cheer and talks to other people going through loss or pain.

She and Craig lead additional youth meetings together and entertain friends for meals or overnight. In addition, Becki keeps up with other activities of their church, does her grocery shopping, cleans house, launders and irons piles of clothes, and mothers that energetic Hayden.

Then—just for exercise—she hops on her bike or jogs a couple of miles on her Canadian crutches. A super-happy week will also include skiing and using her national certification as a handicapped ski instructor to help another disabled person experience the thrill of an outdoor adventure.

God gave Becki an outstanding attitude and physical ability after her amputation. She has open doors into the hearts of many hurting people because of God's work in her. He has given her a fulfilling ministry through her one-on-one contacts, her speaking opportunities, radio and TV appearances, and a variety of magazine and newspaper stories.

However, Becki has had other experiences where God didn't work miracles or give immediate peace. She hasn't always had instant inner healing when she wanted it.

Through all her times—the good and the bad—Becki maintains an openness that reveals she knows she's still "in process." While she is becoming the woman God wants her to be, he is using her to give a charge of joy to those of us around her.

## Chronology of Becki's Life

| | |
|---|---|
| Born in Newton, Kansas | September 27, 1961 |
| Moved to Carol Stream, Illinois | November 1963 |
| Personal commitment to Christ | 1965 |
| Moved to Urbana, Illinois | September 1969 |
| First biopsy | October 21, 1976 |
| Second biopsy | November 11, 1977 |
| Amputation | March 28, 1978 |
| High school Homecoming Queen | Fall 1978 |
| First speaking engagements | Spring 1979 |
| High school graduation (Urbana) | June 3, 1979 |
| First magazine article *(Moody Monthly)* | June 1979 |
| First TV and radio appearances | Fall 1979 |
| Attended Taylor University (Indiana) | Fall 1979—Spring 1981 |
| Moved to southern California | August 1981 |
| Attended San Diego State University | Fall 1981—Spring 1982 |
| Met Craig Sanders | December 1981 |
| Attended California Polytechnic University (Pomona) | Fall 1982—Spring 1984 |
| Married Craig Sanders | June 18, 1983 |
| Graduated Cal Poly, Pomona; B.S.in Recreation Therapy | June 1984 |
| Employed as recreation therapist for the disabled, including St. Joseph's Hospital, Burbank, California | 1982—the present |
| Moved to northern California | July 1986 |
| Hayden Anne Sanders born | October 30, 1987 |

Becki can be contacted for speaking engagements by writing to her at Christian Living Resouces, P. O. Box 3790, Fullerton, CA 92634.

# Notes

### Chapter 2: Happy Birthday, Becki
[1]Dr. Kline later described the tumor this way: "She required left above-the-knee amputation for a low-grade fibrous variety of well-differentiated intramedullary osteogenic sarcoma. This is a special variety of osteogenic sarcoma with a more benign appearance on microscopic examination, but with potential for metastases and mortality. This lesion is described in an article by Doctors Unni, Dahlan et al in *Cancer* vol 40, 1977. This is a very rare lesion with about 30-40 cases in the world literature." (Letter from Dr. Scott V. Kline; Chairman, Department of Orthopedics; Carle Clinic; Urbana, Illinois; July 7, 1986.)

### Chapter 3: I Helped Make That Leg
[1]For the story of Jim's turn-around experience, see pages 299-301 in *Men in Mid-Life Crisis* (Elgin, Ill.: David C. Cook Publishing Co., 1978).
[2]Ibid.

### Chapter 10: God Doesn't Make Mistakes
[1]Joni and Friends, *All God's Children* (Woodland Hills, Calif.: Joni and Friends, 1981), p. 8.

### Chapter 11: A Crisis Is Unfair
[1]"Only You," Kelly Willard and Bruce Hibbard, © 1981, Maranatha! Music, Willing Heart Music (Admin. by Maranatha! Music) and Emmaus Music. All rights reserved. International copyright secured.
[2]Robert L. Wise, *When There Is No Miracle* (Glendale, Calif.: Regal Books, 1977) pp. 42, 44.

### Chapter 12: A Crisis Makes Us Stop
[1]Gordon MacDonald, *Restoring Your Spiritual Passion* (Nashville, Tenn.: Thomas Nelson Publishers, 1986), pp. 29-30.
[2]Ibid., p. 30.

### Chapter 14: A Crisis Reminds Us We Are Temporary
[1]Philip Yancey, *Where Is God When It Hurts?* (Grand Rapids, Mich.: Zondervan Publishing House, 1977), p. 52.